The Unspoken Truth About Essential Oils

Lessons Learned Wisdom Gained

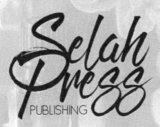

Selah Press PUBLISHING

Stacey Haluka & Kayla Fioravanti

The Unspoken Truth About Essential Oils: Lessons Learned, Wisdom Gained

By Stacey Haluka and Kayla Fioravanti, Certified Aromatherapist
Editor: Venessa Knizley
Cover Design: Stacey Haluka

ISBN-13: 978-0692130957 (Selah Press)
ISBN-10:0692130950

Printed in the United States of America, Published by Selah Press
For information on getting permission for reprints and excerpts, contact: kayla@kaylafioravanti.com

PRAISES

With more people exploring aromatherapy and essential oils it is important to understand they are not a harmless substance. In this book Stacey has been brave enough to share her experience. Not only was Stacey harmed by essential oils, but the damage was perpetuated by individuals that were not trained properly. Kayla helps to clear up some of the many myths that are spread concerning essential oils. This is a good precautionary true story about why you should seek out multiple sources when researching and educating yourself. This is a valuable book for anyone interested in using essential oils. Every aromatherapist should have a copy of *The Unspoken Truth About Essential Oils* to share with their clients, I know I will. *~Anna Pageau–Certified Aromatherapist and Herbalist for humans and animals at Anna's Musings*

Essential oils are wonderful and natural healing substances. However when they are not used properly they can be very harmful. It's time the world understands just how powerful they are! I am so happy Stacey was brave enough to share her story with the world. *The Unspoken Truth About Essential Oils* is so important to the average user. Many people have stories like this but are too afraid to speak up. Thank you for addressing such an important topic! Essential oil safety should always be first and foremost. *~Melissa Clymer–Clinical Aromatherapist, Traditional Naturopath and Herbalist at Sweet Willow Spirit Therapies*

The Unspoken Truth About Essential Oils is a must read! As a professional in this industry I see injuries from essential oils on a regular basis, many of them could have and should have been prevented. I am grateful to Stacey for sharing her story and I believe that together with Kayla's expertise, they will bring awareness to safe essential oil usage and proper education. I am hopeful that this book will reduce these life-changing injuries one copy at a time! *~N. Ruth Nelson–Certified Aromatherapist at DeRu Extracts*

With the increasing popularity of essential oils, the amount of people reporting adverse reactions and injuries is ever increasing. Unfortunately, those that try to share their stories of injuries are often

shunned and attacked…this is why stories like Stacey's are important to share with the general public. I commend Stacey for her bravery in sharing her personal and painful journey. I hope her story will give others the courage to speak up against unsafe essential oil practices.
~*Grant Greene*

This book is such a timely and much needed realistic view of what's really happening in the growing sect of essential oil. Stacey Haluka and Kayla Fioravanti are a wonderful pairing of two women on different plains with a common goal….to inform the public of the real and present unspoken truth about essential oils and the current misguided trends of use and information being widely perpetuated. And in the process, hopefully prevent more people from experiencing life altering events to their health and personal well-being from the misinformed and ill-advised rhetoric surrounding essential oils and the complementary therapeutic modality of aromatherapy.

Sadly, Stacey's experience is not isolated or exaggerated. We in the field of aromatherapy are, unfortunately, seeing and hearing personal accounts of minor to severe injuries and adverse reactions—from misuse and over-use of essential oils, stemming from uneducated guidance—happening far more frequently. Medical advice and usage protocols are being given by masses of people solely trained in sales and "business building" often representing themselves as professionals with extensive education and expertise in health and wellness modalities. But nothing could be farther from the truth. It's now reached a critical point that can no longer be shoved under the rug or denied, though many may try.

Kayla steps up to the plate with her no-nonsense approach, skilled writing and expertise as a long-time qualified aromatherapist to address the many myths, lies, and dangerous practices that have become epidemic in nature. She takes her many years of education, research and experience—pulls on the reserves of the science and art that makes aromatherapy what it really is—and delivers a serious reality check we all can learn from and should heed with respect. Kayla introduces a balance and accountability in regards to these potent chemicals that's both refreshing and eye-opening. Starkly contrasting to what is predominantly seen and referenced in the digital and hard copy world today, her wise words combine research-based evidence with anecdotal experience to bring us front and center without rose-colored glasses, grandiose promises, or claims that blind and redirect the reader from reality.

I encourage anyone who is interested in exploring or currently using essential oils for any reason to get this book and read it with objectivity and consideration for the authors' real-life experiences and hard-earned knowledge. Let it be a word of caution and a truth-filled guide to doing better and being better in your personal journey into the world of aromatherapy. You'll be glad you did. ~Ginger L. Moore– Senior Administrator for Essential Oil Consumer Safety Advocates

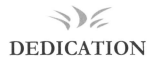

DEDICATION

To all of the people who have experienced a reaction to essential oils, my heart goes out to you. My wish for you is that you will continue to get better every day, in every way. May your healing journey be fast and easy.

To all of the lovely people who have sent me numerous messages of prayers, love and support I am truly grateful for each and every one of you. Thank you from the bottom of my heart for reaching out to me.

To Cindy Nolet and Debbie Cornelius, thank you for your love and support throughout my entire journey.

To Ruth Nelson, Melissa Clymer, Cori Nevills, Anna Pageau, Kristi Martin, Sherry Mandel Harvey and Michelle Castro, thank you! I could not have helped so many people without your dedication, expertise and continued support for the greater good.

To Robert Tisserand and Martin Watt, thank you for your expertise and support. I appreciate your commitment to educate people on proper usage and safety guidelines, as well as your dedication to document people's reactions to essential oils.

To all of you who are currently using essential oils and have had amazing success with them, I am truly happy for you. I wish you continued health in mind, body and soul with the power of plant medicine. I hope that this book will encourage you to expand your knowledge and further your education to learn all that you can about the chemistry and safety of essential oils.

Anita and Scott, I have no words that can express how truly grateful I am for you. From picking me up off of the floor in my darkest hours, to your continued support and encouragement, I honestly don't know if I would be here to write this book if it were not for the two of you.

In light and love,
Stacey

For me, this book is dedicated to all the aromatherapy pioneers who have blazed a path for the rest of us with their passion and dedication. My head is filled with the teachings of Sylla Sheppard-Hanger, Dr. Robert Pappas, Robert Tisserand, Martin Watt, Tony Burfield, Gabriel Mojay, Jeanne Rose, Len and Shirley Price, Marge Clark, David Williams, Salvatore Battagia, Jean Valent and so many more. They have created an incredible resource of experience, knowledge and training that has impacted me greatly and will do the same for generations to come. I am so grateful for all that I have gleaned from them over the years. Above all, I am grateful to the Creator for the amazing design of plants.

Blessings,
Kayla

CONTENTS

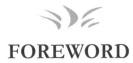

FOREWORD
by Dr. Robert Pappas

Integrity, training, and a dogged pursuit of the truth are the qualities that Kayla Fioravanti has shown in the essential oil industry since 1998. I first started working with Kayla and her husband Dennis in 2003 as a consultant to test the quality of the essential oils that they sold. Over the years we have all developed a friendship based on mutual respect, and a reciprocal desire to share information that is steeped in facts, and as ally's in the pursuit to uncover and disprove misinformation.

I trust Kayla as an essential oil authority. Above and beyond that, Robert Tisserand's Adverse Reaction Report and Martin Watt's Conclusions shared in *The Unspoken Truth About Essential Oils* elevates the credibility of the information in this book to the highest level. Both Tisserand and Watt are pioneers in the essential oil industry that can be trusted.

The Unspoken Truth About Essential Oils retells Stacey Haluka's essential oil injury experience as a representative in a multi-level company. Stacey sought guidance from her sponsors and the company, but was told that she was having a detox experience. In my opinion the detox theory is a desperate attempt to give a positive explanation for any adverse reactions caused by essential oils and is physiologically impossible. Science and Stacey's true story shared in this book thoroughly disproves the detox theory.

If you, or someone you know, uses essential oils this book is a must read. Stacey's story along with the advice shared by Kayla set the foundation for an excellent guidebook to steer clear of some of the common misinformation about essential oils. Kayla backs up her opinions with information from countless experts in the field—myself included. There will be many who disparage this book and the authors because the information in it may contradict the teachings of the companies they are associated with—ignore them. The profits made by the sale of this book pale greatly in comparison to the product sales made by those who would guide you to overuse essential oils.

The Unspoken Truth About Essential Oils will arm readers with accurate information, connect them with true experts, and provide links to resources for future information. Keep an open mind and continue reading if what is shared between these pages contradicts what you have always been taught. If your upline or company that you represent frowns on your reading this book—that's the most obvious sign that you should keep reading. People with nothing to fear will never try to censor information. One can only make informed decisions when information has been gathered from diverse sources.

Essential oils are something I have been passionate about for more than 22 years and with the rapid growth in their use in the USA, accompanied by the over-zealous marketing hype, this will undoubtedly lead to more and more injuries that could have been avoided through proper education. This is why resources such as this book are so important. Ultimately I want people to understand that essential oils are not to be feared, but they are to be respected.

Dr. Robert Pappas—Ph.D. Chemist and independent consultant for the fragrance, flavor, and essential oil industry at Essential Oil University.

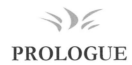

PROLOGUE

I have a story to tell. It is my intention and deep yearning to share this story for the purpose of educating you, the reader, so that you may become more aware of how to incorporate essential oils into your life. It is my hope that by sharing my story you will seek the guidance of a qualified aromatherapist so that you can continue to benefit from the amazing healing powers of essential oils.

At the time of writing this, in March of 2018, I still struggle on a daily basis as the marks on my body remain and flare up from time to time. The experience I want to share with you tested my physical, emotional and mental capabilities to the point where I had completely given up on life. The severe effects of this may be something that I will have to deal with for a very long time.

I have spent a lot of time and money trying to find products that I can use—both personal and household products—that won't make me breakout. It is astonishing to me that the majority of these kinds of products contain fragrance, perfume and/or essential oils, none of which I can use any longer. I also have a difficult time going to some public places or gatherings for the simple fact that everyone is either wearing perfume or essential oils. I have had a few instances where I developed a rash very quickly after simply hugging someone. This has quite a negative effect on me as I love hugging people, but now I often hold back for fear of having a reaction.

I have also spoken with several essential oil experts and have had to unlearn most of what I had initially learned from the multi-level marketing company I was involved in. I have learned that once you have had severe reactions and have become sensitized to essential oils, you will most likely never be able to use them again and may even develop other allergies. I can't even begin to fathom the long-term effects and irreversible damage that has been done to my body, my organs and my immune system from the essential oils, supplements and all of the heavy medications I had no choice but to take—all to counteract something that I thought was the answer to my prayers of finding a holistic solution to help myself and others.

Since I have become sensitized—and even allergic to essential oils—I cannot use them anymore, which saddens me greatly. Even though I have had this horrible experience, I still believe in the healing power of essential oils when used properly and under the care of a qualified aromatherapist.

The chief medical officer of a well-known multi-level marketing company recently made a safety video in which he stated, "There's really no wrong way to use essential oils." However, there are many wrong ways to use them. I would not be sharing my story if there wasn't. Essential oils are very wonderful and powerful, however, they are not meant to be used several times a day, every day, and they are almost never to be taken internally. It is my greatest hope that once you have read this book you will have a greater understanding of just how potent and powerful essential oils are, and that you will use them under the guidance of a qualified aromatherapist or essential oil expert. I want everyone to have a wonderful and profound healing experience with essential oils.

It is my hope that by sharing my story, it will help bring awareness so that others will have a better understanding of what could possibly happen if essential oils are not used properly. Even if you have used them for years and have had no problems, there is still a chance for you to develop a sensitivity to them if you use them too often.

Think about it like this: if someone becomes an alcoholic, there are no signs that they are doing any damage to their body, until many years later they suddenly have liver failure. The same is true for sensitization to essential oils, it can happen at any time and may not show up for several years. I urge you to really pay heed to the information and utilize the resources that Kayla has provided in the second part of this book. It could save you or someone you love from a lot of pain and anguish.

Stacey Haluka

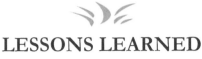

LESSONS LEARNED
by Stacey Haluka

I am lying in bed, preparing myself for another restless night. My body feels like it's submerged in molten lava, my skin is so itchy that I want to rip it apart with my nails and tears are rolling down my face as I say my nightly prayer, "God, please take me in my sleep. I don't want to live anymore. I'd rather die than live another day with this pain and agony. Please take me in my sleep."

Some nights, I would say the prayer silently; other nights, I would yell it out loud, wailing in misery, hoping someone was listening. I would sleep lightly off and on throughout the night, waking up in pain and anguish. When morning would finally come, I would open my eyes in anger that I was still alive and that I'd have to live through another day of agony. I would ask, "Why is this happening to me? Why is my body failing me?" There were so many questions that I didn't have the answers to.

To understand how I got here, I will start at the beginning. It was October of 2014 when I first received my essential oil starter kit from a multi-level marketing company that I will call Pure Essential Oils (PEO). I was over the moon excited, as this was the answer to my prayers. For several years, I had wanted to find an organic and natural solution to help people heal, and, suddenly, I had the answer in my hands. I was going to save the world, or at least anyone who would let me help them. I had done research on the company, it's owners and what their products could do for people. Their sustainability practices, and the fact that they were supporting farmers from all over the world, won my heart over. I loved what I was reading. *This was the company I wanted to work with!* It was with their essential oils that I was going to make a difference and help heal people who had nowhere else to turn.

I began reading the materials that came with my kit and went on-line to complete the recommended website trainings so that I could learn everything possible about these little bottles of gold. I was surprised when I read that PEO essential oils were so pure that I could even take them internally. I knew that aromatherapists say that you should not take essential oils internally, but I was told by my upline that their training was outdated. "Aromatherapists must not be using essential oils that are as pure as PEO's." This was a whole new world for me, as I had used essential oils occasionally for years, but none of them had ever claimed to be pure enough for internal use. None of them said they were therapeutic grade.

I watched a training video supplied by PEO that stated the majority of essential oils on the market are diluted with synthetics. After that, I threw out every single bottle that I had previously purchased from the health food store. PEO not only said that I could use their essential oils topically, internally and aromatically, daily, they encouraged their usage *several* times a day. They stated that I only had to dilute the essential oils if I had sensitive skin. I pondered, "I don't have sensitive skin, so I can apply them neat (undiluted), *right?*"

I began experimenting with the PEO essential oils from my kit. I applied different ones to my body several times a day, took them internally and diffused them throughout my home most of the day and beside my bed at night. Who wouldn't want lavender diffusing beside them while they sleep? I was in essential oil heaven!

I spent several hours every day learning as much as I could on PEO's website and through their "university training." I've always been someone who wants to be educated in what I'm using, especially if I'm going to recommend and sell it to others. I wanted to know everything I could about these therapeutic grade essential oils. The information I was learning was fascinating! I learned the best places on my body to apply the essential oils for total absorption, like the bottoms of the feet and along the spine. I learned that diffusing essential oils was the safest way to get them into your system. I learned that these essential oils could also be used on children, babies and even animals! I learned that these essential oils could help with almost any ailment or illness that is out there. Like I said, I found gold!

After all my PEO research and training, I felt confident enough to begin teaching classes. PEO had made it so easy, as they provide training scripts for teaching classes. I also purchased a training kit complete with a DVD to show the class, along with samples of orange essential oils to hand out for people to try. PEO suggests we get people to put a drop in their hands and rub them together, hold their hands over their face to breathe the scent in and then take the essential oil internally. This was a great way for people to experience all of the different ways they could benefit from essential oils. I was determined to get these seemingly miraculous essential oils into their hands, just like I had been taught. Whatever the ailment, I had an oil for it!

Late in November of 2014, I was in the backyard when I noticed a small rash on my forearm. I had no ¡ rash had come from, so I went inside the house and applied ⸗ ⸗ *undiluted* tea tree essential oil, since I had read that it was supposed to be good for skin rashes. I had used another brand of tea tree oil several times in the past, but I saw this as an opportunity to try PEO's brand.

I applied tea tree essential oil again later that evening before I went to bed. The next day the rash was still there, so I applied more tea tree to my arm several times throughout the day. This continued to be my daily practice, however, the rash wasn't getting better, in fact, it had gotten worse and had begun to spread up my arm.

I began asking others who sold PEO for recommendations. I asked my upline directly about it in our private Facebook groups. Every leader has their own Facebook group, so there were several that I belonged to. I asked if it was possible that I was having an allergic reaction to the essential oils?

I was told, "No, you can't be allergic to the oils, PEO's website states that essential oils do not contain allergens, nor do they contain any protein molecules, so in turn, they cannot cause a true allergic reaction."

It was recommended that I try applying essential oils that were good for the skin such as lavender, geranium, lemongrass and myrrh. They also said, "when in doubt, use frankincense." I began making up concoctions with these essential oils and organic coconut oil that I would slather on my skin several times a day throughout the month of December.

It was around this time that I had also began taking three different supplements from PEO in a Healthy Life Pack which included a Cellular Vitality Complex, a Micronutrient Complex and an Essential Oil Omega Complex, which included clove, frankincense, thyme, cumin, orange, peppermint, ginger, carraway and chamomile. The Healthy Life Pack stated that it was formulated to provide targeted levels of essential nutrients and powerful metabolic factors for optimal health, energy and longevity. Everyone I had asked about these supplements said that they were "life-changing," and that the best part was that they even came with a 30-day money back guarantee! I couldn't go wrong; they sounded like the exact thing I needed!

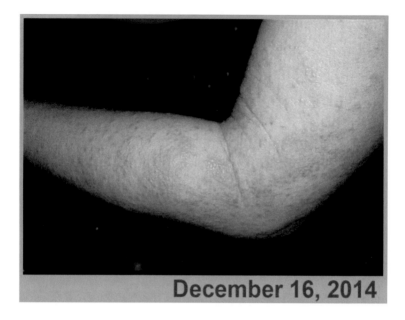

December 16, 2014

By January, the itching had become unbearable, and the rash had started to spread to my left leg and the back of my neck.

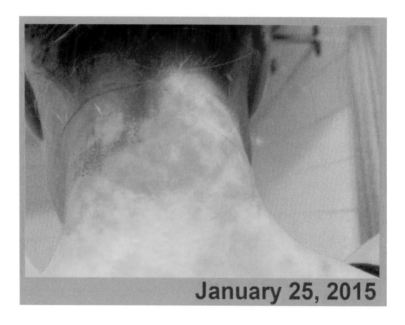

January 25, 2015

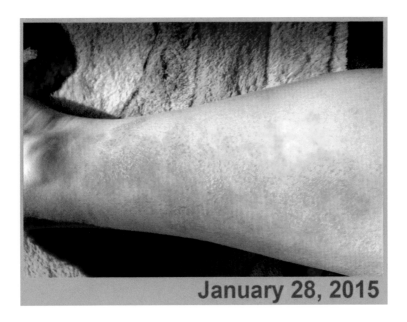

January 28, 2015

I will note here that I had never applied any essential oils to my forearm, neck or leg prior to the rash developing. I couldn't figure out where this rash was coming from. I hadn't really introduced anything new to my life, as I had been using essential oils occasionally for several years, and I had never reacted to them before. I had to find out what was going on, so I called PEO's corporate office directly, however, they said they couldn't help me, and that they were unable to answer any of my questions. I once again reached out to my upline and to our Facebook groups, as it seemed that was the only place I would get any help. The information that I learned was astonishing, I was having a detox reaction! *A what?*

I was told by a woman in my upline, "A detox reaction. When you begin taking essential oils internally, they are cleansing your body, organs and tissues, right down to the cellular level. One of the sure signs of this is when your body breaks out in a rash because this is how the body will get rid of toxins, through the skin, which is called a detox reaction. This is a good thing. Now that you know what it is, you just have to keep using the concoctions you have made on the actual rash and continue taking the Healthy Life Pack supplements. Don't worry, it should only take a few months to completely detox."

A few months? That seems like a long time to be itchy, but if this is what it takes to completely detox my body, I'll deal with it. Later on in

January, I had an upset stomach, which I assumed was part of the detoxing. I applied a digestive blend to my abdomen to help calm it. The next day I woke up with a rash on my abdomen. This was the first time that a rash appeared on the area where I applied the essential oil.

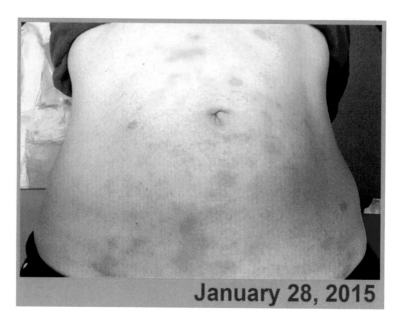

January 28, 2015

Since it was on my abdomen, I assumed it was simply another detox reaction. Once again, I searched for PEO protocols for skin rashes, trying different combinations of the essential oils and applying them to my skin several times a day. I believed in the healing powers of these amazing essential oils so much that I knew there had to be a combination that would be right. I just had to find it.

This is the point when the itching and burning was completely unbearable, and my nightly prayers began. I couldn't bear anything touching my skin, including clothes. The only thing I could wear was a soft onesie, which I pretty much lived in every day. I wanted to rip my skin apart. My body started swelling up, my limbs were so swollen that I couldn't bend my arms fully and I began having a fever and severe diarrhea.

I couldn't take it anymore. My body was breaking down physically, emotionally and mentally. In February of 2015, I went to my family Doctor. I left the office with a prescription for a strong steroid in pill form and a very strong steroid cream to apply to my skin. My doctor also gave me paperwork to get blood work and urine samples taken. All tests came back perfectly fine! I was told that there was nothing wrong with me, so my doctor told me to keep taking the medications and wait it out.

A few days later on a Sunday, I ended up going to the emergency room, as the fiery pain and itching was just unbearable. I felt like someone had locked me in a room with mosquitoes, wasps and fire ants and left me there. The doctor I saw told me that there was nothing he could do, and that I needed to go back to my family doctor. He gave me a prescription for a strong anti-histamine to help with the itching and burning and to try to keep me comfortable. *Comfortable?* There was no "comfortable" at this point, and I was literally beginning to go out of my mind!

I hid in my house, wearing my onesies, secluded in my pain and misery. I didn't tell anyone what was going on with me—I didn't know what was going on with me! I distanced myself from friends and family members. I didn't know how people would react if they saw me. I didn't know if I was contagious, and I was in no shape to even leave the house unless I absolutely had to. I was hiding from the world, suffering in silence and spiraling into a deep depression. I still couldn't eat anything without it going right through me, and as a result I ended up losing almost 15 pounds in less than two months. I was skin and bones.

Come March, I had completed a couple of rounds of the detox with the Healthy Life Pack supplements. The rash had improved due to the steroids I was ingesting and applying to my skin, although I wasn't feeling much better overall. I was lethargic, depressed and felt like I had a very bad flu. I continued to take the PEO supplements and incorporated another essential oil blend that was supposed to protect the body and cells from oxidative stress and improve cellular health. This priming blend consisted of clove, thyme, orange, frankincense, lemongrass, savory and niaouli. After having to take steroid medication, I thought that my system was toxic again and I needed some extra help.

In the middle of March, I had a pimple forming on my face so I applied frankincense to it as I was told it was one of the most mild, yet effective essential oils. The next day that spot was still red, so I put frankincense on it again. The following day, it was worse, and I began to panic! *Not my face! This can't be happening!* I applied lavender to my face. Again—let me remind you that I was not in my right mind at this point. The redness was spreading and my face began swelling up.

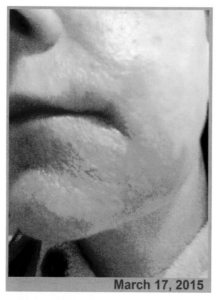

March 17, 2015

Within a few days, I felt some fluid seeping out of my face. I kept applying lavender; I was frantic, something had to work! However, it got worse, and my entire face swelled and become very red. The leaking from the open sore became so bad that I had to tape a gauze bandage to my face 24 hours a day because it seeped constantly and wouldn't stop.

After getting out of the shower, the crusty skin would peel off and leave my face raw, red and painful.

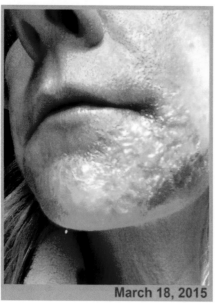

March 18, 2015

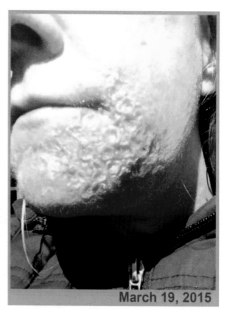

March 19, 2015

I was looking at myself in the mirror in tears. I can't keep going on like this. *I just want to die!* This was when it struck me—there had not been a rash on my face until I applied the frankincense. It was then that

I realized the essential oils were the actual cause of the rash. That was when I decided to stop everything. I stopped using the PEO essential oils and supplements completely.

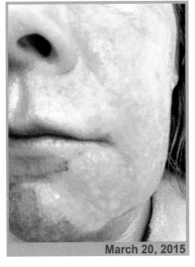

March 20, 2015

Within a day after I stopped applying the oils to my face, the leaking began to subside. The open sore began to heal, and the swelling and redness began to subside. My face had almost completely healed within about ten days after I stopped using the essential oils and taking the supplements.

Although my face had healed after I stopped applying the essential oils, the rash on the rest of my body remained. *Now what do I do? Will this ever end?* My friends had always commented on how beautiful my skin was, and now I couldn't even look at myself. Prior to this time, I had been a vegetarian who was generally in good health. I'd never had any major ailments or illnesses. I had always sought out holistic nutrition and supplements, and very rarely took any medications unless absolutely necessary. *Why was my body failing me now?* There were so many questions with absolutely no answers.

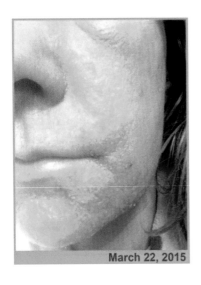

March 22, 2015

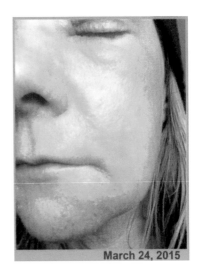

March 24, 2015

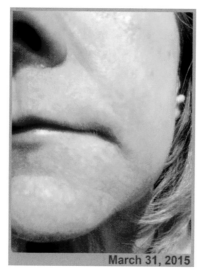

March 31, 2015

Throughout this whole ordeal if and when I left the house, it was only for brief periods of time, and only after I had lathered myself in anti-itching cream. I didn't let anyone see me unless they were helping me heal. I became severely depressed and could not see the light at the end of the tunnel. I was miserable, in pain and on edge.

It was in April of 2015 that I decided I wasn't going to hide and suffer in silence anymore. I contacted the top of my upline, one of the Canadian Founders of PEO who I will refer to as Donna. I emailed Donna to tell her what had happened to me, along with photographs that I had taken throughout the last few months. She stated that she wished I would have told her sooner as she would have told me to stop using the essential oils and taking the supplements. I thought to myself, *Hmmm, has this happened to someone else before?*

Donna then referred me to the PEO's Product Safety Department. Throughout a short period of time, I had several email exchanges and phone call conversations with two gentlemen from the product safety department.

During these interactions, I asked, "Had this ever happened to anyone else? Has anyone else ever had a serious reaction from using the essential oils?"

They responded, "We cannot answer that ma'am."

However, I noticed that at the bottom of his email it stated, "For health emergencies for which you believe a PEO product is a contributing factor, please discontinue the use of the product immediately. If symptoms persist, contact a medical professional."

If there had never been any other severe reactions, why would this information be part of the signature in his email?

I also asked the safety department if there was a plan for PEO to implement a training program for everyone in regards to proper safety and precautionary use of their products.

Their response was, "We are not sure ma'am, however I can forward this question to the department in charge of that."

I responded, "If I had thought for one second that these essential oils were the cause of what was happening to me, I would have stopped using them immediately, which would have saved me a lot of pain and suffering."

Instead, I was brainwashed into thinking that someone could not have an allergic reaction to these "therapeutic grade" essential oils. I believed that my rash was a good thing, as my body was expelling toxins. This belief caused me to suffer greatly.

I requested to speak with the Chief Medical Officer, who I will refer to as Dr. Falls. I told them I was desperate for answers and needed to talk with him since he was purported to be PEO's expert on essential oils. I was told that Dr. Falls was currently out of town. However, the gentleman from the safety department, assured me that my information would be forwarded to him. I never did hear back from him, and every time I spoke with, or emailed, the two men from the product safety department, I would ask if my information and photos had been forwarded to Dr. Falls. Each time, they assured me that he had my information and that I would hear from him when he had time.

On May 22, 2015, I wrote an email to the PEO safety department which included, "I am also wondering if there have been others who have reacted so severely? Is there something in the works to create more awareness about what can possibly happen? I do not want to see anyone else go through this. From the beginning I had taken it upon myself to learn about PEO and the products, and with that I was researching and using every suggested protocol that I came across to try to ease the rash, the pain, itchiness, swelling and oozing. What I ended up doing was making it worse all around, but I kept trying different combinations of oils that were suggested. Had I had any inclination that they were the actual cause, I would have stopped immediately. I would really love to see some guidelines or training put in place." And, "Also, I am going to ask you to please forward my emails to Dr. Falls once again. I am asking for help as I would like to get to the bottom of this."

I never did get any answers to any of my questions, and I began to feel like I was becoming a nuisance to them. During one conversation with PEO's product safety officer, I was put on hold so he could speak to Dr. Falls' secretary.

After a few minutes, he came back on the line to tell me, "Yes, Dr.

Falls has looked at my information, however, he is out of town at the moment. His secretary has assured me that you will hear from him when he has time."

In all honesty, I don't know if my information was ever sent to him, however, if it was, I can't believe that someone in his position would ignore helping me after seeing my photographs and hearing my story. It was extremely disheartening to say the least, and I felt even more alone and frustrated than I did before.

As time went on, my rash continued to flare up every now and again, and I had no choice but to use the steroid creams on it. Although it wasn't quite as bad as it had been, it was still very itchy, raw and painful. Upon seeing my naturopathic doctor, and after she reviewed my blood test results, I was advised that my immune system had been compromised due to the stress that all of this had had on my body. It was also possible that there was some internal damage due to taking essential oils orally.

In June of 2015, I went to see an allergy specialist. He advised me to stop using the essential oils, which I had already done at this point, and once again, I was given a different medication in cream form.

In December of 2015, I went to my family doctor after another flare up and left with another prescription cream.

In February of 2016, I went to see a dermatologist. She believed my rash was caused from something my skin had been in contact with. For confirmation, she took a biopsy from my leg, stitched me up and gave me yet another medical cream. The biopsy left a scar on my leg, and the results showed that it was indeed contact dermatitis.

She referred me to another allergy specialist to have an allergy patch test done. In June, I went to the Allergy and Dermatology Department Patch Test Clinic at McMaster Hospital in Hamilton to have the skin patch test applied. I brought several of PEO's essential oils with me, and I asked the doctor if he could test me for reactions to them. Unfortunately, the allergy patch test is a standardized test, and he could not test them on me. However, the essential oils of tea tree and ylang ylang were included in the standardized test. After wearing the patches for four days, I returned for the results, which confirmed that I was highly allergic to both tea tree and ylang ylang essential oils.

Through heavy medications and stopping the use of essential oils my rash would go away for periods of time, however there were times throughout 2016 and 2017 that I would still breakout. Currently, I am scared to touch anything for fear that I will go back to that dark place that I was in not so long ago.

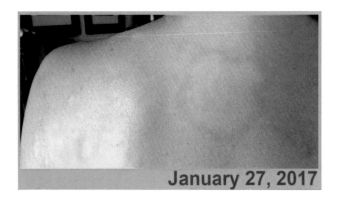

January 27, 2017

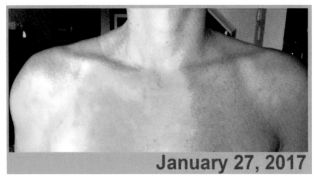

January 27, 2017

For well over a year now, I still have several white spots on my body where there appears to be a permanent loss of pigmentation. This has caused me to feel ashamed of the body that I once loved so dearly. I wonder what people will think when they see me in a tank top or a bathing suit. *How do I explain all of this to them? They're just essential oils after all. They're pure and natural; they couldn't possibly be harmful to anyone, or could they?*

In July of 2017, I decided that I was going to go public with my experience and no longer suffer alone. I felt that I had to share my story so that I could help bring awareness to others of the potential dangers of using essential oils. Since I went public, I have had several people contact me from all over the world reporting that they have also had serious reactions to PEO essential oils.

Some of the stories people have shared with me have broken my heart, as I completely understand what they are going through. Others were in the midst of their pain, going to doctors and allergy specialists trying to figure out what was going on. It still breaks my heart that so many people are having serious reactions due to misinformation about safety and protocols provided by PEO.

After I went public, Donna—one of the Canadian Founders of PEO that I had previously reached out to—contacted me. I spoke with her on the phone. "Stacey, why didn't you tell me about this? I would have helped you."

If she could have seen my face she would have witnessed the shock that registered. I couldn't believe what I was hearing.

I responded, "Donna, I *DID* come to you with this. I emailed you my photographs and spoke with you on the phone about what was happening to me. Don't you remember?"

She replied, "Ooops, I guess I forgot, sorry."

Sorry? She forgot? What? How could someone in her position forget something like this? I honestly couldn't believe what I was hearing. She then asked me if I had contacted PEO's product safety department and if they helped me. I told her I'd had numerous conversations via email and phone with them, however, I didn't get the help that I had been looking for.

"What would you like to see changed?" she asked.

"I want PEO to hire qualified aromatherapists to provide people with proper safety and protocol information. I want PEO to provide proper training for everyone who sells their products and for their staff. I want people to be aware of the possible dangers by PEO sharing my story," was my response.

"Well how much should we tell people without scaring them off?" she asked.

I responded "All of it! They should know everything. If people were more aware of what could happen to themselves or their children, they would understand just how powerful essential oils are and would hopefully use them like medications—only when needed."

Donna didn't agree with me, and so the conversation ended there. It saddens me that she was more worried about scaring people off than helping people understand the potency, power and possible dangers of misuse.

It also saddens me that PEO has been negligent and irresponsible about providing proper training to their downline in regard to safety, precautions and possible dangers. When a new person enrolls and receives their first order, there is no training that is received, other than an email with a few links and three brochures.

It is incomprehensible to me that a company that seems to care so much, could care so little about the severity of what could happen due to improper information. Essential oils are extremely powerful and should be treated as such. Distributing them to the public for healing without any information is like a doctor providing you with a prescription without a list of possible side effects or how to take the medication, and then refusing to help you when your body reacts to it.

What if this were to happen a child? To someone's baby? I honestly don't think that a baby would be able to live through this kind of pain and suffering. I believe that the mother who thinks she is helping her child would forever blame herself, and all because she thought she was doing the right thing. Essential oils are very powerful and strong and should ALWAYS be diluted and used with caution. PEO has no one to contact for support or questions regarding safe usage and protocols, so people turn to each other in the Facebook groups for answers. I have documented several cases where people posted questions regarding reactions and rashes in the Facebook groups of my uplines, and some of the responses and suggestions that are posted are ludicrous! These people are NOT the experts!

I do not want anyone else to ever have to go through what I have gone through. It was for this reason, I asked PEO to implement a thorough safety and precautionary training program that every current salesperson would have to sign off on. Every new person that enrolls would receive this training, in the form of a booklet, in their initial order, along with a DVD that would include protocols and answers to: how to test each EO for a reaction, what to do if you have a reaction, how to use the oils safely, possible interactions, etc. I also asked PEO to re-train their call centre to better assist people with their questions and to employ essential oil experts to help people who have questions. To my knowledge, none of this has been implemented.

Back in 2015, when I had requested a meeting with Dr. Falls to help me understand why all of this had happened to me, I had also wanted to ask what he recommended going forward to help me get better and boost my immune system. I was exhausted from trying to figure this out. The doctor's I'd seen had not been much help in regard to providing me with answers or solutions, as they were only looking at things from their limited perspective and knowledge of essential oils. I've recently discovered that Dr. Falls is actually a chiropractor, not a

Medical Doctor, although his title is Chief Medical Officer of PEO. In a recent video, Dr. Falls indicated that, "one of the things I have responsibility for, of course, are all of the adverse events that occur with essential oils." I will admit that this breaks my heart to hear as he did not take any responsible action in responding to me. I would have liked some resolution and peace of mind, however, I have yet to hear ANY response to my requests.

It was only when I began speaking with qualified aromatherapists that I began getting answers. Such as, when I had stopped using essential oils on my skin and taking them internally, I hadn't stop diffusing them. It was only from the experts that I discovered why I was continuing to react and have break outs—it was because I was still diffusing them beside my bed all night long! I had no idea that diffusing essential oils was still harming me!

I had the pleasure of speaking with Roxanne Benton of Patriot Botanicals who also became sensitized to essential oils. She stated, "I'm injured from essential oils—as in, I can't use them topically pretty much at all. I had an aromatherapy massage with a technique that uses undiluted essential oils nearly three years ago about a week before my back surgery. I rashed out so badly that I thought I may have to postpone the surgery. Luckily, we didn't have to. Even on my feet—bottom or tops—well-meaning people (before I figured out WHAT the heck was going on) would oil me up—and in the next day or so—BAM. Itchy, red rashes. Oy! I can't be in the room when Helichrysm is bottled or my face swells up just from the fumes. HOW CRAZY IS THAT?! I found that one out the hard way. Gah! It makes me itchy just thinking about it....and I don't even LIKE Helichrysum!" (Roxanne Benton 2018).

It was this statement that got me thinking about public diffusing. There are way too many people out there casually diffusing essential oils in their stores, at wellness expo's, yoga classes and even in schools. Public diffusing is negligence and could cause someone great harm! You do not know the medical history and body chemistry of every person that will come in contact with the diffused oils.

I also began to wonder if this may be the reason why the rashes on my body flare up from time to time. I have become sensitized to so many different essential oils that it's possible that simply smelling them, whether through diffusion or from someone wearing them, can cause me to have a reaction. I know for certain that I have reacted on a few occasions simply by hugging someone as an itchy rash broke out on my arms within a very short period of time after.

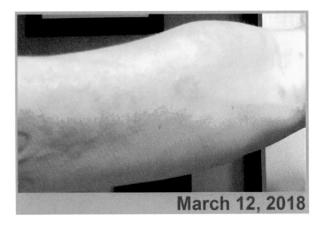

March 12, 2018

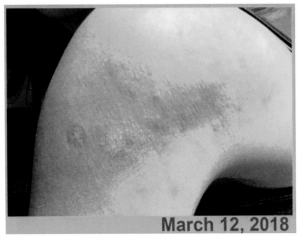

March 12, 2018

I have heard of children having a hard time breathing, feeling nauseas and getting severe headaches because their teacher was diffusing in the classroom. The same can apply to constant diffusing in your own home because children and animals are very sensitive and are at a higher risk of having ill-effects. Please don't let your children become sensitized or cause harm to your family pet. You will never forgive yourself. For these reasons, I beg of you, please stop diffusing essential oils in public! What you do in your own home is your choice, but hopefully by the end of this book, you will begin to choose differently.

When I'd initially enrolled with PEO, I truly believed that I had finally found what I had been searching for, for years—a holistic answer to people's health concerns. I have not used any antibiotics, steroids, or other medications for many years—except the occasional over-the-counter headache medication. I have always tried to find a natural solution to any health issues and have wanted to create awareness and help others do the same. I thought PEO was a dream come true! I have heard so many amazing stories of healing that people have had with essential oils, however, I must say that my experience was beyond horrific. I truly would not want anyone else to go through this pain on any level. Please don't be someone who says, "this won't happen to me," because it can happen to you; it can happen to anyone. It doesn't matter how healthy you are, if you don't have sensitive skin or if you've been using essential oils for years. I truly hope that this book will give you the nudge you need to learn about the chemical composition of essential oils, along with the proper safety protocols to implement them.

If you are someone who has had, or is currently having, a reaction, I pray that you find some peace, strength, support and comfort. I would also urge you to report your reaction. You will find the links to do so in the Resources section of this book.

My Evolving Journey

Since going public with my story in July of 2017, more and more people have become aware of the possible dangers of essential oils. I have had several people reach out to me, asking me what I did to get better, however I cannot give them a definitive answer. I am not an aromatherapist or a doctor, and there doesn't seem to be any experts who can help someone who has become sensitized to essential oils. It would give me great satisfaction if I could give them relief from their pain and suffering—if I could wave my magic wand and make it go away. The truth is, I can't. I am simply figuring all of this as I go along. I have invested a lot of energy, time and money on several therapies, vitamins, minerals and supplements...you name it, I've probably tried it. Each time I try something new, I pray that it will work, that I will finally be completely healthy again and have my life back.

In September of 2017, I still felt like I wanted to leave this planet. I was tired of simply existing and exhausted from this long and arduous journey. This was not how I imagined life would be, this was not a life worth living. However, I made a decision that if I was going to stay here I was going to start making some serious changes—so I gave myself six months to expand my life and embrace new knowledge. Since that time I have joined a mastermind group and have become certified in four different modalities and therapies. My path is unfolding before me and I am trusting that the Universe has my back.

Recently my naturopathic doctor suggested I work on lymphatic drainage, and it really seems to be helping. I have been seeing my osteopath for lymphatic drainage, and have been dry brushing and rebounding on my mini-trampoline daily. I will continue to find comfort in my meditation and spiritual practice, spending time in nature, with my dog and supportive friends….I also highly subscribe to 'wind therapy' on my motorcycle.

This experience has taught me just how strong and resilient I am. I am focused on rebuilding my life and my business, which gives me great satisfaction and purpose. I will continue on this journey of enlightenment, expansion, healing and growth….and I WILL WIN!

Namaste

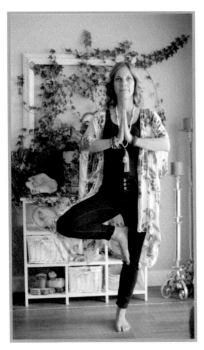

"Be the change you wish to be." – Stacey Haluka

ADVERSE REACTION REPORT
by Robert Tisserand

This is not a case where we can say that a specific oil caused a localized skin reaction. It can be characterized as a systemic allergic reaction, in the sense that it spread and also worsened much more than in most people.

It should be emphasized that this case is not typical in its severity, extent and duration. However, lessons can be learned:

1. It's likely that the application of undiluted Tea Tree oil exacerbated the initial rash. The topical application of undiluted essential oils does generally increase the risk of an adverse skin reaction, especially with Tea Tree oil.

2. The problem was made worse by continued application of essential oils, often undiluted, in the mistaken belief that this would be helpful, and that the oils could not possibly be the cause of the problem.

3. Taking oral supplements long-term that contain a significant number of essential oils, in combination with intensive topical application, likely contributed to the eventual systemic reaction.

4. This person's skin reaction was not "detoxification," in the sense that the liver needed help from essential oils to "detox." In fact, the progression of symptoms suggest that the body was reacting to the cumulative effect of long-term essential oil use, internally and topically. Taking other supplements, and applying topical medications, may have added to the burden on the liver.

5. In cases of an allergic reaction this severe to multiple oils, complete avoidance of all essential oils is advisable. Eventually, this is what happened, leading to a significant reduction in symptoms.

Robert Tisserand—Expert in Aromatherapy and Essential Oil Research, and co-author of *Essential Oil Safety*.

Used with Permission: Tisserand Institute. *Adverse Reaction Database.*
http://tisserandinstitute.org/safety/adverse-reaction-database/#home/adverse-reaction-report-detailed-view/5996e998b34c36291baf0f98/

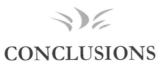

CONCLUSIONS
by Martin Watt

In the case specific to Stacey Haluka, it is my opinion that she was harmed due to the company not providing accurate safety information during the training of their distributors. Instead, she was advised that people only get reactions from adulterated essential oils and that her body's reaction was due to detoxing. Both of these concepts are total nonsense and 100% false. Had she received proper training and education from the company or their agents, the extensive trauma she experienced would never have happened.

Since she had a previous experience prior to this being atopic (an allergic predisposition), she should never have used essential oils on her skin, however, she was not made aware of this. This all goes back to the fact these multi-level distributors are not trained properly by the parent companies, and, therefore, they are not asking the correct questions before advising people on what essential oils to use.

The lack of safety advice provided by these multi level companies angers me. There is sound data on the dangers of certain essential oils going back over 50 years. Data that is known to reputable essential oil suppliers.

I just hope Stacey's skin will heal without any scars or loss of skin pigmentation. She now needs to be very careful when encountering essential oils, as she may be permanently sensitized to some of them. My best advice to her is do not use any essential oils on the skin, even if they are in body products.

I get very sad and annoyed when I see cases like Stacey's. I have spent over 25 years trying to educate people about essential oil safety and even created a trade safety manual, which was sold internationally. Too many people are being harmed by essential oils because of lack of education and the belief that they are pure and natural. They, therefore, believe oils can do no harm, which is completely false!

Martin Watt Cert Phyt (Herbal Medicine)
Used with Permission: **www.aromamedical.org** (Please do not share without prior written consent from Martin Watt)

WISDOM GAINED

by Kayla Fioravanti, Certified Aromatherapist

I am an accidental aromatherapist. I discovered essential oils when all else had failed when my son got ringworm. We had tried over-the-counter (OTC) drugs and prescriptions to clear it up, but it kept growing. Since I was partly raised while living overseas, I had learned to go to the apothecary to find natural cures. So, I headed to the tiny, local health food store, which was the closest thing I could find to an apothecary. The store clerk had nothing to do but stand in the book aisle and read books with me in search of a natural remedy. Everything we read pointed to tea tree essential oil as the cure to ringworm.

At that time, our family was on a very tight student budget, so I bought the smallest bottle of tea tree essential oil available and headed home to see if my eleven-dollar investment would work. Much to my surprise, within three days the ringworm was completely gone. In addition, I had expected the tea tree to cause allergic reactions because I am allergic to fragrances, but I had no problems. Because of that combination of events, I became very intrigued about this thing called aromatherapy.

Before that encounter with tea tree essential oil, I had always just assumed that aromatherapy was one of the foo-foo fluffery esoteric things out there in the market. When I thought of aromatherapy, I envisioned the incense burners that make me take the long way around the hippy haven stores that line Hawthorne Avenue in Portland, Oregon.

With my new found interest in the healing benefits of essential oils, I went to the local library and checked out every book they had on aromatherapy. After I read those, I put in a request for all the aromatherapy books available in the state to be sent to my local library. Once I started digging into the science of essential oils, I was fully addicted to learning. In 1998 I started researching and studying to become a certified aromatherapist. I have been in love with, intrigued by and in awe of the power of essential oils ever since.

Because I am obsessive in my research, I even borrowed books that were not available in the library from a friend who was in a multi-level essential oil company. I read each book from cover to cover, but I could not ignore the fact that the methods of application, not only conflicted with all the other books—but literally seemed to spit in the face of every bit of safety advice of the other authors from Germany, England, France and the United States.

For the next sixteen years, I worked in the aromatherapy industry as a buyer, supplier, manufacturer, aromatherapist, perfumer and educator without saying a word about my fundamental disagreement with what the popular essential oil multi-level companies were teaching. And then one day, when a friend was advised by a representative to give their young son undiluted vetiver essential oil to drink—I broke my silence with a blog post that went viral teaching the safety rules that the multi-levels were not teaching. I could no longer silently co-exist while people were injured all around me due to unsafe practices.

That blog post, in 2014, still attracts countless readers, and, as a result, my inbox continues to be full of emails from injured people. The worst are the panicked parents seeking advice when their two-year-old is screaming in pain in the middle of the night with welts forming where they applied undiluted essential oils on their children at the advice of their upline. Calls to the upline were answered with the detox theory.

Essential oils, when used properly, are amazing and wonderful. I agreed to work with Stacey on this book because I want everyone to be able to use essential oils for a lifetime. I hate that Stacey has been denied that opportunity and has suffered so greatly. I use essential oils every single day, and I cannot imagine my life without them. I sincerely want the same for others. It is from that place that I share the following information. I hope to shine a light onto the myths, half-truths and outright unsafe teachings.

Myths About Aromatherapists

Could it possibly be true that all aromatherapists have out of date information? Or that as a whole, the industry is under educated? Can you imagine the organization it would take for there to actually be a conspiracy between aromatherapists—to keep all the essential oil business to ourselves by disagreeing with the multi-level organizations on the topic of safety?

The reality is that aromatherapists are in a constant state of learning. I have been in the aromatherapy industry for twenty years and have never rested on the knowledge I gained twenty years ago. I don't know a single aromatherapist who has. The pursuit of knowledge among people who are passionate about aromatherapy is universal. The key is to get information from a variety of sources. Never, ever stick to information from one school, one business organization or one aromatherapist. Read information that contradicts what you have been taught with an open mind. You will see throughout this book that I give references to a variety of people in the aromatherapy industry.

So could it be a lack of education? Entire organizations are dedicated to the further education, training, research and development of the aromatherapy industry. The school choices to become a certified aromatherapist are extremely varied and accessible. There are associations, national and international meetings, tele-seminars, books, videos and so many more resources that aromatherapist are able to further their education.

But again, could it be that aromatherapists just want to keep all the business to themselves? According to Grand View Research, "The global aromatherapy market size was valued at USD 1.07 billion in 2016 and is projected to witness lucrative growth over the forecast period. Rising awareness about therapeutic uses of essential oils has led to the growth of the aromatherapy market" (Grand View Research 2017). Surely, there is enough business to go around without needing to disparage other essential oil companies. There is, quite frankly, enough business to go around for independent aromatherapists, without the need to take out the competition.

Often, aromatherapists have been accused of being scaremongers because they insist on teaching safety that is in direct contradiction to what the multi-levels teach. This idea could not be further from the truth. Aromatherapists love essential oils. We want people to experience the amazing healing benefits of essential oils. We simply want them to do it safely. Teaching people to respect the amazing potency of essential oils should never be considered fearmongering.

The Myth of the French Method
So, could it be true that aromatherapists simply, as a general rule, adhere to a single school of aromatherapy that is different than the multi-level companies? I'd be rich if I had a penny for the number of times someone has told me that they drink essential oils because they practice the so-called "French Method" of aromatherapy. Let's explore

that reasoning. Many believe that aromatherapy diversified into four basic groups in recent years:

1. In England, the use of aromatherapy is from massage, an external and safety-conscious approach.
2. In France, the practice of aromatherapy comes from a medicinal, internal and experimental approach.
3. In Germany, aromatherapy is approached from a medicinal and research-oriented point of view.
4. The United States practices aromatherapy through massage, external use, esthetic, and eclectic approaches.

The reality is that there are only methods of application and not "schools" of aromatherapy as many suggest. Gabriel Mojay addressed this topic in an open letter to Sylla Sheppard-Hanger, Director of the Atlantic Institute of Aromatherapy entitled, "British vs. French Aromatherapy—a myth…or a smokescreen?" On June 29, 2014.

"Dear Sylla,
I'm not sure I would call this business over 'British vs. French Aromatherapy' a 'myth,' as such—more of a ploy by MLM [multi-level marketing] distributors to distract people from the fact that they are overwhelmingly unqualified to recommend or administer the intensive/internal methodologies commonly associated with the 'French' approach they lay claim to.

My concern is that they aren't even equipped with adequate knowledge to safely direct people to use essential oils via dermal methods of application, which they simplistically brand as 'British'—let alone via the oral route. Their invention and promotion of potentially skin-sensitizing applications, such as 'raindrop' and 'aromatouch,' makes this glaringly obvious.

In a nutshell: the so-called 'French' and 'British' labels are being used to mislead and mystify.

Their use of these labels misleads by giving the impression that they represent contrasting therapeutic systems, as for example between orthodox and natural medicine—whereas they are no more than simplistic, somewhat nationalistic, ways of distinguishing between different sets of methodologies…methodologies that, properly understood, belong to a single, integrated therapeutic discipline: **Aromatherapy.**

Their use of the 'French' and 'British' labels mystifies by obscuring the crucial difference between the methodologies they represent—**which is the training required to safely administer them** …rather than the countries some continue to associate them with.

Doctors can prescribe pharmaceutical drugs because they have completed the necessary training to correctly and safely do so—not on the basis of merely asserting the proposed benefits of those drugs. Simply hailing the superiority of the so-called 'French' style of Aromatherapy does not give a person the moral right to administer internal/intensive methodologies without even basic training.

Look at the training and examinations physicians are required to undergo to prescribe pharmaceutical drugs. Given their pharmacological potency, why should essential oils be treated so fundamentally differently? It doesn't make sense.

Exponents of such sales tactics make bizarre statements to justify their contempt for proper, accredited education, such as, "The British are more interested in 'aroma' than they are in 'therapy'—an affront to all those Aromatherapists who work tirelessly, and often voluntarily, in palliative and cancer care, in particular."

The same author claims that "The French school emphasizes that aromatherapy is safe and can be practiced, with common sense, by anyone whether trained in the healing arts or not." Why then is it illegal in France for anyone other than a physician or registered pharmacist to therapeutically administer essential oils? His argument doesn't add up.

About one thing, however, he is correct: 'The British school **[though I prefer myself to call it the International Ethical school]** emphasizes that essential oils have their hazards and is best practiced by trained, certified professionals.'…Yes, sir—and you will find that the same conviction is part of the bedrock of every other branch of orthodox and natural medicine.

With warm wishes from your devoted colleague,
Gabriel Mojay
London
[Feel free to share… no need to ask, thanks.]"

Medical use of aromatherapy is completely prohibited or restricted in much of the United States. Beware of anyone telling you that they are simply practicing the French method of aromatherapy when they suggest internal usage of essential oils. The French field of Aromamedicine is extremely scientific and includes thorough assessments by qualified practitioners using an aromatogram.

The aromatogram was developed in 1969 by Maurice Girault, based on the 1949 research article "Methods for comparing the antibacterial activity of essential oils and other aqueous insoluble compounds" by Schroder and Messing (Jennifer Peace Rhind). An aromatogram is a test used to determine the antibacterial activity of an essential oil against a pathogenic sample from an infected patient. This is done by culturing a sample of blood, urine, feces, saliva, vomit, discharge, skin or another infected biological material in a petri dish. Single note essential oils are then placed around the perimeter of the dish to test the reaction and effectiveness against the microbes over a 24-hour period at 37 °C (98.6 °F). The center of each petri dish contains a disk of filter paper saturated with a different essential oil. The diameter of the clear zone, where no bacteria is able to grow, determines the efficacy of each essential oil against the pathogen. Based on the results, a combination of essential oils may be encapsulated and prescribed for treatment by medically qualified doctors with relevant training. That is a far cry from your neighbor telling you to just drink essential oils or put them in a capsule without any knowledge of your medical history or any training in aromamedicine.

It is also important to hear that not every French doctor has the training to practice aromamedicine. Absolutely no American doctors have the relevant training, even if they have joined a multi-level company and are selling essential oils using the credibility of the medical degree as a sales tool.

In October 2017, Robert Tisserand and Hana Tisserand traveled to Grasse, France to attend the 18th Phyt'Arom Conference to learn directly from the source about the so called, "French School." In a blog post, entitled "Grasse Phyt'Arom 2017–what we learned in France about French aromatherapy," on the Tisserand Institute website, Hana Tisserand wrote, "Robert and I were really looking forward to learn more about the French approach. What we totally did not expect was to find that they are doing almost exactly what we have been advocating for, and that aromatherapy in France is changing. We listened to speaker after speaker talking about proper dilution, the importance of safety. Some even advocated for the preference of topical application and inhalation over ingestion." One of the most telling quotes from the blog post came from Dr. Guilhem Jocteur who is a pharmacist and educator. "When we [Robert and Hana] asked him if putting essential oils in water to drink was an option, his reaction was as swift as surprised: *Mais ca ne mélange pas!* (But they don't mix!)" (Hana Tisserand 2017).

My view is that essential oils should not be consumed or used undiluted without, at the very least, proper training and certification, the use of an aromatogram, a known medical history, knowledge of essential oil chemistry, understanding of drug interactions and a thorough understanding of sensitization. Certified Aromatherapist Melissa Clymer of Sweet Willow Spirit Therapies asked an excellent question when she wrote, "Stop with the 'I have been ingesting xyz for x years and I'm fine.' HOW DO YOU KNOW? You cannot see the damage these highly concentrated substances are doing to your organs, or tissues" (Melissa Clymer 2018).

A common argument is that certain essential oils are Generally Recognized as Safe (GRAS), so it is safe to consume them. However, comparing essential oils used in the food industry to consumers dropping essential oils in their water is like comparing apples to oranges. "Did you know that 1 tablespoon of mint oil will flavor 135,000 sticks of chewing gum?" (Peppermint Jim's). Ruth Nelson explains, "1 tablespoon is about 15ml or 300 drops if you are using the 20d/ml ratio. This is about 0.002 parts of 1 drop per piece of gum" (Ruth Nelson 2018). The English Aromatherapist states, "These GRAS guidelines are measured in parts per million! To give you an idea, 1 part per million is roughly equivalent to one drop in 50 liters (more than 150 cans of Coca-Cola). When we consume them in manufactured food and drinks, we're ingesting minuscule amounts. This is completely different to adding whole drops to our glass of water at home! (FYI, you are not 'diluting' the oil in the water—oil and water don't mix!)" (The English Aromatherapist).

Quality of Brand XYZ versus Everyone Else
Could it be that aromatherapists simply do not have the access to unadulterated essential oils? I do not dispute the quality of the essential oils that any company sells. There is a myth widely spread that brand XYZ has the only essential oils in the whole wide world that are pure enough to be safe for consumption. *Wait! What?* The logic of that goes

out the window immediately if you know at all how potent a pure unadulterated essential oil actually can be.

Essential oils are the most concentrated form of any botanical. It takes an estimated one pound of any given plant to create one drop of essential oil; however, some essential oils require much more than a pound of product per drop. For example according to Jeanne Rose, it takes 60 rose buds, to produce one drop of rose absolute (Jeanne Rose 2006).

So is it true that brand XYZ has the only therapeutic brand of essential oils? To this day there is not a certifying force or standardization of therapeutic grade essential oils. The implication put out by some companies that there is such a grade or standardization is pure fiction and brilliant marketing. This marketing ploy creates a dependence on that supplier for a particular "grade" of essential oil that is perceived to only be available from them. The perception is true, because the grade was randomly set by the supplier and cannot be followed by another supplier. There is no regulatory agency that defines, monitors or enforces these marketing "grades" and "standards." There is little to no difference in the chemical make-up of essential oils sold with these various marketing ploys to the essential oils sold by reputable essential oil companies.

Could it be true that aromatherapists are settling for adulterated essential oils and that is why we don't suggest consuming them? Many aromatherapists have incredibly educated noses, know how to read essential oil analysis reports, have long established relationships with their suppliers and want nothing but the best essential oils for themselves, their family and their clients. Aromatherapists are definitely not settling for adulterated essential oils or being duped.

Unfortunately the injury reports that we are seeing are increasing at a rapid rate because the myth continues to spread that company XYZ has such pure essential oils that they are safe to consume.

The Myth of Allergies
A common myth about essential oils is that since they are natural, you can't be allergic to them. However, there is no such thing as 100% hypo-allergenic because of the way the human body reacts to things that it perceives as a foreign invader.

Skin allergies are very common, but allergies can impact any area of the body. A skin allergy reaction can appear in the form of a rash, welt or hives. These inflammations of the skin may be in isolated patches or in general areas. In order to have an allergic reaction, you simply need to have been exposed at least one time to a substance, at which time, your body identifies it as a foreign invader. The next time you're exposed to that substance, your body sends out the troops to protect itself, and, suddenly, you have an allergic reaction. Your body has an exaggerated immune response. The same substance will cause absolutely no reaction in non-allergic people because the body sees the substance as harmless. Many times, an allergic reaction shows up on the skin whether it was caused by topical, aerial or internal exposure to an essential oil.

An allergy is the body's immune system rejection of a substance— that substance can be natural or unnatural. The body does not differentiate between the two. If it was even possibly true that natural products were never the cause of allergic reactions, how do you explain nut allergies? Mold allergies? Hay fever? The list goes on and on of completely 100% natural things that people are mildly or severely allergic to.

An allergic reaction is caused when the immune system sees a substance as a foreign invader. In reaction to the foreign invasion of allergens, the body sends T-cells—a group of white blood cells—out to fight. In skin allergic reactions, this causes redness and irritation. Your risk of developing an allergy isn't necessarily related to the natural or chemical composition of a substance, but instead it is related to your parents' allergy history.

Some people believe that since essential oils contain no proteins that they cannot cause allergic reactions. This is best explained on the Tisserand Institute page in a blog post entitled "New Survey Reveals Dangers of Not Diluting Essential Oils," in which Robert Tisserand writes, "Some essential oil constituents, such as cinnamaldehyde, can cause allergies because they are haptens. This means that they are 'protein-reactive'; they bind with proteins in the skin. More specifically, they bind with peptides (short chains of amino acids) on the surface of Langerhans cells, and the Langerhans cells then migrate to local lymph glands, where the peptide-allergen complex is presented to T-lymphocytes. Antibodies are then created, and the next time the same hapten contacts the skin, an allergic reaction is almost inevitable" (Robert Tisserand 2017).

The skin is not the only organ susceptible to allergic reactions. Allergies can manifest in mild, major and life-threatening ways. The body can react with a cough, sneeze, eczema, contact dermatitis, hives,

runny nose, asthma, digestive upset, dizziness and even anaphylaxis.
At any time in your life, you can develop an allergy to any thing on earth. No one is completely immune. Over use and excessive exposure can increase the likelihood of someone eventually developing a sensitivity or allergy.

Sensitization

Now, let's talk about the very real topic of sensitization. This one breaks my heart because, in most cases, sensitization is totally avoidable. Most people who use properly diluted essentials oils will not develop sensitization. One of the huge factors in sensitization is dosage. An essential oil diluted at 1% is significantly less of a dose than an undiluted application of 100% essential oil. Some of the other factors that increase your risk of sensitization include your genetic predisposition, rate of absorption, general health, age and frequency of exposure.

In case you are not familiar with the term sensitization—or believe that aromatherapists are fear-mongers who made it up—here are a few definitions:

Miller-Keane Encyclopedia and Dictionary of Medicine, Nursing, and Allied Health: exposure to allergen that results in the development of hypersensitivity.

Farlex Partner Medical Dictionary: Immunization, especially with reference to antigens (immunogens) not associated with infections.

Mosby's Medical Dictionary: Reaction in which specific antibodies develop in response to an antigen. Allergic reactions result from excess sensitization to a foreign protein.

Improving your chances of avoiding sensitization is as easy as properly diluting essential oils. Also, know the chemistry of essential oils—know when to dilute them further than the standard application.

Because essential oils are able to enter the body through percutaneous absorption, I highly recommend conducting a patch test and always using diluted essential oils. A patch test can be performed by applying 1-2 drops of diluted essential oil on the forearm or back and then apply a bandage. The patch should be left on for 48 hours if there is no initial irritation. If at any point during the patch test there is any irritation, the bandage should be removed, and the area should be cleaned with soap and water. Please do not assume that only topical application of an essential oil can cause an allergic reaction. Martin Watt explained it best in a personal communication regarding this book, "It only takes a few molecules to get into the superficial layers of the skin in order to trigger an allergic reaction" (Watt 2018). Stacey experienced continued allergic reactions, even after ceasing internal and topical usage, from continuing to diffuse essentials oils.

One may not always know right away that they are having an allergic reaction. In the article "Sensitization—What Is It and How To Reduce The Risk" on Aromatherapy United, Ginger Moore wrote, "Delayed allergic reaction typically occurs with the first exposure to a substance but usually presents with no symptoms or with only a slight or barely noticeable effect to the skin. Subsequent skin exposure to the same material, or to a similar one with commonalities, will produce a more severe inflammatory reaction with each exposure's symptoms being worse than the last. These will present as inflammation, blotchiness, redness, itchiness, rash or may resemble a heat or chemical burn on the skin. Some individuals may also experience pain with a moderate to severe reaction. Again, these symptoms are usually localized to the area of contact but could happen anywhere on the body where no contact between the skin and the substance has occurred" (Ginger Moore 2016).

Moore goes on to explain, "The problem with dermal sensitization is that once it occurs with a specific essential oil, the individual is most likely going to be sensitive to it for many years to come and perhaps for his/her lifetime. The individual may possibly never be able to have topical exposure to that essential oil or ones in the same family ever again" (Ginger Moore 2016). This is precisely the predicament that Stacey finds herself in now.

In a series on essential oil safety matters, Beverley Hawkins writes, "Sensitization reactions can also take the form of inflammation, breathlessness, nausea or headache. It is actually possible to become sensitized to any essential oil. Sensitization to an essential oil can happen through overuse of any oil, and an interesting fact is that Lavender (*Lavendula angustifolium*), the essential oil with the reputation of being one of the most versatile and safest essential oils around, is the one that most therapists have become sensitized to. This happens mainly through overuse of the oil, a good reminder that we should not just use the same oil or blend of oil day in and day out but we should change our blends around on a regular basis" (Beverley Hawkins).

It is critical to understand that once sensitized, one may find themselves unable to use a large variety of essential oils, cleaning products, personal care products and more. According to Martin Watt, "It should be pointed out that sensitization only occurs to specific chemicals in an essential oil, not to the whole oil. So, for example, if someone is sensitized to orange oil, they are probably reacting to the d-limonene or its breakdown chemicals. That means they will react to ANY other oil containing appreciable amounts of the same chemical/s, and there are a lot containing that one" (Watt 2018). Many cleaning products contain d-limonene, and since regulations on household cleaning products do not require an ingredient list, the consumer is left to find new products through trial and error. Grapefruit, lemon, orange, lime, bergamot, niaouli, peppermint, nutmeg, mandarin and lavender essential oils, just to name a few, all contain d-limonene.

What can you do to help ensure that you never find yourself unable to use your favorite essential oil? The key is to dilute, dilute, dilute. I may sound like a broken record, but properly diluted essential oils greatly reduce your risks. I will provide a chart with dilution rates for specific uses of essential oils in this book.

Less is more when it comes to essential oils. Many are taught to use essential oils in their food, drinks, diffuser, inhaler, neat on their skin, improperly diluted on the skin and in every single aspect of their lives. While that does sell a lot of essential oils, it also increases your exposure and puts you at risk. A perfect storm is created when people use essential oils topically, diffuse them in the air and also take them internally.

Some people would rather read the basic facts in plain English, and others want the science. For those who want the science Tony Burfield and Sylla Sheppard-Hanger wrote an article entitled, "Sensitization Revisited Again," which explained, "During the sensitization process many of the chemicals present in the essential oil will penetrate the epidermis. After biodistribution, certain of the components may be biotransformed by the xenobiotic and P-450 enzymes in the skin to haptens (which we can think of as allergens). This transformation may also be induced in certain instances by UV light. Once formed the haptens react with nucleophilic residues on proteins forming antigenic sites. The immune system then swings into action and a response is generated" (Tony Burfield and Sylla Sheppard-Hanger).

Burfield and Sheppard-Hanger explain further, "At a more complex level, such as might result from considering essential oil biotranformations, several haptens may compete for a limited number of sites on the protein (antigenic competition). The relatively higher concentration of the least strongly bound haptens may cause a feedback mechanism to operate within the enzymes producing the hapten, which may alter the sensitization profile of the mix. The rate of release of absorbed substances from the epidermis, and the concentration at the protein site will also affect hapten-binding" (Tony Burfield and Sylla Sheppard-Hanger).

Now let's go for the plain English version. Kelly Taylor of Cassia Aromatics gave an excellent example when she said, "WOULD you drink a chemical degreaser or an oven cleaner? If not, then you would not want to drink lemon essential oil, because the active ingredient, d-limonene, is the *exact same component* that you can buy with this ingredient for chemical, industrial degreasers, caustics, and oven cleaners" (Kelly Ann Taylor 2018). I know many people do not want to believe that the naturally occurring d-limonene in degreasers, and many cleaners, actually comes from citrus fruits, but it is true.

Taylor goes on to give a clear and concise explanation that should be required reading. She explains, "Think about it. Or, look at herbalism. In terms of 'strength' it goes like this.

1) tea
2) emulsion
3) decoction
4) tincture then and finally
5) essential oil

Exponentially does not mean 4x4=16. It means 4 to the fourth power or 4x4x4x4 = an exponent of the whole herb counterpart. One drop of peppermint essential oil is equal to 28 cups of tea. Exponential means 'to the power of.' Exceedingly strong" (Kelly Ann Taylor 2018).

Melissa Clymer, CA goes onto say, "The next time you reach for that essential oil to take it internally, please remember that there are other, better, safer and more gentle ways to use it. Or, look at the herbal equivalent. Just because you can do something, doesn't mean you should" (Melissa Clymer 2018).

There are also options to get a whole citrus fruit in your drink without using essential oils. Mediterranean-style lemonade is made by food processing a whole lemon with ice and your choice of sweetener. Delicious and safe. You can also just wash your citrus fruits and then add whole slices into your water. My personal go-to is to add lavender, rose or orange blossom distillate water to my favorite lemon-aid recipe. The possibilities with distillate waters, which are a by-product of making essential oils, are endless.

A Bit About Contact Dermatitis

After much pain and far too long, Stacey was eventually told she had contact dermatitis. According to the Mayo Clinic, contact dermatitis is, "a red, itchy rash caused by direct contact with a substance or an allergic reaction to it. The rash isn't contagious or life-threatening, but it can be very uncomfortable. To treat contact dermatitis successfully, you need to identify and avoid the cause of your reaction. If you can avoid the offending substance, the rash usually clears up in two to four weeks" (Mayo Clinic). Common symptoms of contact dermatitis include a red rash, swelling, burning, and tenderness. The skin can be dry, itchy, cracked or scaly. It can also include bumps and blisters that ooze or crust over" (Mayo Clinic).

The most common form is irritant contact dermatitis. The Mayo Clinic explains, "This non-allergic skin reaction occurs when a substance damages your skin's outer protective layer. Some people react to strong irritants after a single exposure. Others may develop signs and symptoms after repeated exposures to even mild irritants" (Mayo Clinic). For those who are not allergy prone this can be an alarming bit of news. According to the Mayo Clinic when you experience allergic contact dermatitis, "You may become sensitized to a strong allergen such as poison ivy after a single exposure. Weaker allergens may require multiple exposures over several years to trigger an allergy. Once you develop an allergy to a substance, even a small amount of it can cause a reaction" (Mayo Clinic).

The cure is the same whether it is irritant contact dermatitis or allergic contact dermatitis—avoid all contact with the substance.

Detox Theory

Another common myth that Stacey encountered was the idea that the reaction she was having to an essential oil was really her body detoxifying. Your body reacting to undiluted essential oils is not detoxification! It is most commonly a chemical burn, allergic reaction or inflammatory response. Unfortunately, people are injuring themselves right and left with the belief that the pain, swelling, rash and even blisters are the result of detoxification. It is not. The detox theory in aromatherapy, unfortunately, is not the answer to why you may be having a reaction. Trust me, I wish that the detox theory was a fact and not fiction. The Detox Theory has been disproven on many levels. Many aromatherapists long believed that essential oils could detox the body, however, that was never viewed as anything beyond sweating out toxins—and not a way to explain away rashes, burns and injuries.

According to Merriam Webster Dictionary, detoxify is, "(a) to remove a harmful substance (such as a poison or toxin) or the effect of such from (b) to render (a harmful substance) harmless" (Merriam Webster Dictionary). There are six organs the body uses to eliminate waste and detoxify the body: the liver, kidneys, lungs, lymphatic system, digestive system and skin. A toxin is technically any foreign substance. According to toxicologists a, "Toxic agent is anything that can produce an adverse biological effect. It may be chemical, physical, or biological in form. For example, toxic agents may be chemical (such as cyanide), physical (such as radiation) and biological (such as snake venom)" (European Commission).

A basic simplified explanation of how the organs eliminate toxins can help you understand why detoxification is the wrong term for these adverse reactions. The liver changes the chemical makeup of toxins. The kidneys filter toxins out of the blood through urine. The lungs eliminate toxins by removing them as gases and sometimes phlegm. The lymphatic glands filter infectious agents and produce white blood cells. The digestive system can forcefully eliminate toxins through vomit or diarrhea. And the skin acts as a barrier to keep toxic substances out, but also works to eliminate toxins via sweat.

In a blog post entitled "Essential Oils and the Detox Theory," Kristina Bauer states, "The detox theory in aromatherapy poses a challenge as it suggests that the body's attempt to alert the user to a possible adverse reaction is actually a sign of a positive (detoxification) response. In many ways, the detox theory contradicts conventional thinking about what adverse reactions are—and how they should be addressed—by framing a potential adverse reaction as a favorable response." Bauer goes on to say, "To really drive a detoxification response, an essential oil would have to directly engage with the body's elimination systems" (Kristina Bauer 2015).

Dr. Robert Pappas of Essential Oil University makes one of the best plain English arguments about the detox theory in his debunking myth series. In "Essential Oil Myth #6" he says, "Let's just think about this logically for a second. Let's imagine you rub poison ivy on your skin and you get a really bad rash. Is that just your body detoxing? Of course not. Come on people, if you get a rash or burn from putting something on your skin it's because it's IRRITATING YOUR SKIN" (Dr. Robert Pappas). If you think logically about his example, it is clear that the poison ivy is the foreign invader and the reaction is your body attempting to protect itself from said invader.

Dr. Pappas goes on to say, "And if you are using the term detox reactions to refer to the sweating out of toxins, well think again. The old 'sweating out' toxins myth cannot apply since it's physiologically impossible. This is because toxins (skin cell debris, bacteria etc.) lodge in the pores of plosebaceous units and not in those of sweat glands. A rash or burn from an essential oil is basically your skin screaming at you, "hey, stop that and stop it now!' " (Dr. Robert Pappas).

The withdrawal symptoms of an alcoholic quitting drinking cold turkey, which is a true detoxification process, does not include blisters, rashes and burns on the skin. As the body rids itself of alcohol, often at toxic levels, there are not adverse skin reactions other than sweating.

The detox theory does not hold water no matter what direction you try to spin it. If your liver truly was detoxifying from undiluted topical application or internal usage of essential oils, why would a toxin that had been transformed by the liver result in a rash, burn or blister? It would not. Further, if it really was working like they said it was, why would the adverse reactions get worse over time when the body should be ridding itself of said toxins? Shouldn't it result in a more mild reaction?

Understanding inflammation may further explain why the detox theory is false. The dictionary definition of inflammation is, "a localized physical condition in which part of the body becomes reddened, swollen, hot, and often painful, especially as a reaction to injury or infection" (English Oxford Living Dictionary). The body wants to warn the brain that a stimulus is harmful—inflammation is an attempt to tell your brain to stop using the harmful stimuli so that the body can start to heal itself. If you are experiencing inflammation of any kind in response to aerial, topical or internal usage of essential oils, heal thyself by removing the usage.

The Myth that You Are an Anomaly
Stacey asked PEO repeatedly if she was the only one who had a bad reaction to essential oils. Sadly, she is not alone. The reports of adverse

reactions have been sky-rocketing with the increased popularity of the multi-level companies. Unfortunately, there is a veil of secrecy in many multi-level organizations. Stacey encountered the attitude that allows it to spread when Donna asked her, "Well, how much should we tell them without scaring them off?" I truly believe that education is not scary. Teaching people to understand the extraordinarily diverse and varied chemistry of essentials can only empower people to respectfully use essential oils.

The 2016 American Association of Poison Control Centers report is a good indicator that the improper use of essential oils is on the rise. There were 20,109 poison control cases in 2016 involving essential oils. This landed essential oils in the list of the "Top 25 Greatest Rate of Exposure Increase" of poison control reports (American Association of Poison Control Centers 2016).

Some of the cases in the Aromatherapy United Injury report for 2017 are staggering in their long term implications for the injured parties. One report from January 14, 2017 from some who used essential oils topically, diffused and internally usage reads, "I introduced my mother to essential oils, with the same unsafe application methods as I had been taught by MLM companies. My mother experienced the same rash I did, only hers was full body, and she was eventually hospitalized for an anaphylactic reaction. She had to be on strong steroids for a long time. She underwent allergy testing with a doctor, and is now seeing a naturopathic doctor trying to undo the damage to her body that was done by misuse of oils. It has been over a year since her ER visit, and her body is still not back to normal" (Aromatherapy United 2017).

The report that required medical intervention from a person who used essential oils orally which was made on February 1, 2017, "Underwent colonoscopy and endoscopy in January 2016 (approximately two months after stopping ingestion, side effects were continuing). Results indicated that the lining of my esophagus and stomach had been eaten away" (Aromatherapy United 2017). The personal testimony on the same report reads, "I trusted the advice given by my upline as it was what was recommended by the company (and it was someone I had known for several years who was dealing with severe health issues in her own family). I was dealing with severe mental health issues at the time and was not having any luck with traditional treatments. Essential oils were marketed to me as a natural, safe alternative that would have miraculous effect on my issues. I feel like I was not only given harmful recommendations, but that I was also taken advantage of while in a very vulnerable state. Not only did oils not provide the implied miracles, they caused physical harm that had led to considerable medical expense and issues that I am still dealing with over a year later" (Aromatherapy United 2017).

A highlight of the symptoms the 2017 Aromatherapy United report include: numbness, elevated heart rate, redness, burning, stomach pain, heart palpitations, shortness of breath, reflux, diarrhea, blisters, throat closed requiring epi-pen, welts, burning sensation, anaphylactic reaction, severe kidney pain, urinary retention, severe bladder pain, itchiness, children crying in pain and clutching stomach, nausea, toxic neuropathy, hives, chemical burns, eye irritation, panic sensation, sore throat, gastric upset, pins and needles sensation from head to toe, blisters and ulcers in mouth, tightening of the throat, 2nd degree burns, felt high/drunk, anxiety, shacking, dizziness, unusual heavy menstrual bleeding, sweaty, hot, body on fire, pupils dilated, felt like body was on fire internally, vomiting, oozing skin, weight loss due to chronic symptoms, headache, inflammation, confusion, extreme fatigue, loss of bladder control, slow heart rate and low blood pressure, miscarriage (Aromatherapy United 2017).

Medical intervention and long term consequences for those in the 2017 report include: newly developed multiple chemical sensitivities, unable to use essential oil(s) any longer, considerable short and long term medical expenses, diagnosed with urinary retention and interstitial cystitis, linx surgery required to damaged esophageal sphincter, sensitization, multiple emergency room trips, chemical burns, sensitive skin, huge immunological response, compromised immune system, multiple appointments with specialists, hormone disruption, as well as short and long term required medications (Aromatherapy United 2017).

Believe it or not, most cases are never reported anywhere. Of the hundreds of emails I received in 2017 from injured people, I only recognize one on the injury report. That means that despite being prompted to report—hundreds did not report—and I am only one aromatherapist among thousands getting emails from injured people.

In the resource section of this book, I have provided you with sources to find information about reported injuries, as well as a list of other consumers who want to learn how to safely and effectively use essential oils. Don't be afraid to truly learn the power and chemistry of essential oils outside of the multi-level companies.

What to Do When Injured

When an injury occurs from the use of essential oils:

1. If an essential oil causes dermal irritation, apply a fat such as vegetable oil, coconut oil, olive oil, butter or margarine to the area affected to dilute it. Repeat as needed. If you do not feel relief, seek medical attention. If you do feel relief try washing the area with soap and water. Add more carrier oil if using soap and water increases the dermal irritation.

2. If a child appears to have consumed an essential oil, contact the nearest poison control unit and seek immediate medical attention. For identification purposes, keep the bottle for emergency workers. If an adult is experiencing any symptoms (pain, dizziness, burning, vomiting, irregular heartbeat, elevated blood pressure, severe headache or migraine, reddening, swelling, pain, blistering of the mouth, throat or esophagus, respiratory distress or other alarming adverse reactions), seek medical attention.

3. According to Robert Tisserand, if an essential oil gets into your eyes, the standard treatment is copious irrigation with a saline solution for 1-2 hours. Initially, contact lenses should not be removed (Peate 2007). Fatty oils (carrier oils) have also been suggested as an appropriate first aid treatment for this, though the advantage of saline is that the eyes can be continually flushed, and this is less easy with fatty oil (Robert Tisserand 2013). I would add that you should seek medical attention if you do not have significant relief, as an ocular chemical burn is serious.

4. If you are having a reaction to aerial essential oils, exit the room you are in or step outside for fresh air.

After the Crisis Is Over Report the Injury:

1. Report any essential oil injury to the Atlantic Institute of Aromatherapy and the Tisserand Institute.

2. Report the injury to the FDA. You can use several resources on the FDA website including: *Your Guide To Reporting Problems to*

the FDA, Report Unlawful Sales of Medical Products On The Internet, Consumer Complaint Coordinators–Report A Problem or Medwatch Online Voluntary Reporting Form.

3. You can report a claim to FTC using *File A Complaint With The FTC.*

4. If you are experiencing any problems using any brand of essential oils, especially if they advocate internal usage or undiluted application, please report the problem to whatever brand you are using.

5. Report any poisoning to Poison Control.

Many injuries could be avoided with proper research. The Internet is one source of aromatherapy information, but it is not the gold standard. Anyone can put up a blog, create a social media following and declare themselves an expert. In today's publishing world, the same is true with published books. The burden of proof rests on the consumer and the aromatherapy practitioner to source accurate, safe and dependable information about essential oils. No one should depend solely on the word of one person or organization. A variety of books, research papers, websites, experts and sources should be used to learn about essential oils. When you finish reading this book, I highly suggest picking up another, and another and still another. Become a perpetual student of aromatherapy.

There are multiple sources of dependable information. On Facebook, I recommend following: Essential Oil Consumer Advocates, The Unspoken Truth About Essential Oils, Robert Tisserand Essential Training and Essential Oil University. I'd be personally thrilled if you also followed my Facebook page, Ology Essentials.

Topical Application

Dilute, dilute, dilute. I cannot express enough how important it is to dilute essential oils. One of the clearest explanations of why essential oils need to be diluted comes from Robert Tisserand, "The essential oil in a bottle is 50-100 times more concentrated than in the plant, and safety issues apply to essential oils that may not apply to the whole plant or herbal extract" (Tisserand Institute, Safety Pages). Think about that—50 to 100 times more potent than the plant. That is a significant number.

Although our skin is mostly waterproof, it is still permeable to water, lipids, water soluble solutions and other substances which have small molecular structures and low molecular weight. In aromatherapy, molecules of essential oils applied to the skin pass through the skin's epidermis and are carried away by the capillary blood circulating in the dermis. The molecules of essential oils are then taken into the lymphatic and extracellular fluids. From there, the therapeutic components of the essential oils are broken down and used by various parts of the body.

The human body takes the most vital properties of appropriately applied essential oils, and it uses those properties to bring itself into balance and into a healthier state without side effects. After the essential oils perform their healing functions, they are metabolized and eliminated with the body's other waste.

Nothing beats a great aromatherapy bath, as long as you add something to solubilize the essential oil into your bath water. Any basic science class will teach you that oil and water do not mix. Essential oils will float on top of the water if you drop them into a bathtub or even mix them in salt. My favorite option is to add the essential oils to a carrier oil and then add them to salt or directly into the tub.

Even the mildest of essential oils can burn without a carrier oil. How do I know? Well, let me tell you about the time that a tiny drop of rose absolute burned my skin in the tub. You see, I had an itty-bitty dropper, and I could not get the last drop of rose absolute out of the dropper. I didn't want to waste this precious drop, so I tossed it into the tub for later use. I forgot about the dropper when I turned on the tub water that night. Even when the subtle scent of rose filled the bathroom—it didn't remind me to add some carrier oil. I dropped my entire body into the hot bathwater and quickly came back out with my skin on fire and bright red.

If you don't want to use a carrier oil there are a few alternatives that can help emulsify the essential oil into the bathwater including: Polysorbate 20, Solubol, Sulfated Castor Oil or a surfactant based product such as bubble bath or shower gel.

Adding essential oils to a carrier oil or lotion is a great way to apply them diluted to your skin. As a general rule of thumb, adding 4-5 drops of essential oil to every one ounce of carrier oil creates a product with 1% essential oils. Varying dropper sizes and opinions will result in your finding this advice to range from 3 to 6 drops per ounce being equal to a dilution rate of 1%. My math comes from using a dropper to painstakingly measure 480 drops of essential oil into a 1 ounce container. The math on that is 4.8 drops per ounce, which is why I suggest rounding down to 4 or up to 5 drops per ounce to be at 1%.

> Use four to five drops of essential oil
> per ounce of carrier for 1% dilution rate.

Aerial Inhalation

Essential oils can be diffused into the air through a variety of methods, including a diffuser, room spray, body mist and even perfume. Essential oils have tiny molecules, which disperse into the air and enter through the nose. When inhaled, the scent molecules reach the olfactory epithelium, which consists of two groups of twenty-five million receptor cells each, located at the top of the nostrils, just below and between the eyes. Odors are then converted to messages, which are relayed to the brain for processing. Inhalation provides the most direct route to the brain. Inhalation is very useful for respiratory symptoms and is as easy as sniffing drops on a tissue or cotton ball.

The average person takes about five seconds to breathe—two seconds to inhale and three to exhale. During an average year, we breathe 6,307,200 times. With every breath, we smell. The human body is capable of registering and recognizing thousands of different smells. The sense of smell is ten times more sensitive than the sense of taste. Our ability to distinguish different smells is incredibly precise, but it is almost impossible to describe a smell to someone who has never experienced it. Response to smell only takes 0.5 seconds, as compared to 0.9 seconds to react to pain (Fioravanti).

Using diffusers has become extremely popular. This can be a good and bad thing. It is good because people are replacing chemical ladened room fresheners with natural essential oils. For those of us with allergies to fragrance oils, this is a huge win, but you must keep in mind that increasingly growing populations of people are now allergic or sensitized to essential oils.

In private spaces, remember less is more. One to two drops per one hundred square feet is plenty. And just as you would not clean with bleach multiple times per day, you do not need the strongest most antiviral essential oils diffusing every single day. When it comes to diffusing at night, having something with a sedative property when you are falling asleep is fine, but it isn't necessary to have it running all night long. Reduce your exposures whenever possible. Cindy Rumpf Novack suggests using hydrosols mixed with water in a 1:1 ratio for two hour period of times as a safe diffusing alternative.

> Use one to two drops of essential oil
> in a diffuser per one hundred square feet.

Public spaces are not really the appropriate place to share your enthusiasm for essential oils. This is especially true when it comes to schools, nurseries and day cares. Essential oils are natural medicine, and you do not know the health history, allergies and sensitivities of a given population. Also many of the essential oils that I have come across being diffused in classrooms are simply too strong for the respiratory systems of many students. Unless you are trained in essential oil chemistry you may miss some big warning bells. For instance, Eucalyptus is not safe for children under the age of three. However, I have smelled it wafting from the church nursery and read posts from moms putting it right on their baby's feet!

In the article, "Risk vs. benefit: using potent antimicrobial essential oils with children," Lauren Bridges wrote, "Although some essential oils may be potent antimicrobials, does the way they are currently used preserve the integrity of our children's health? There may be cause for concern, for three reasons. One, the most potently antimicrobial essential oils also tend to be the most risky in terms of adverse skin reactions (Tisserand & Young 2014). Two, although there is not much evidence so far of bacterial resistance to essential oils, it is almost inevitable that this will eventually happen. And three, though essential oils are often touted as 'immune boosting,' there is almost no clinical evidence to support such claims, and in the case of young children, enthusiastic use of essential oils may actually inhibit normal immune development" (Lauren Bridges 2017).

In her conclusion, Bridges says, "With effective options available that are less risky than the 'big guns,' using clove, cinnamon, thyme thymol, oregano and similar oils for every little sniffle is tantamount to dumping a gallon of water on a match to extinguish a flame that could have been snuffed out with a little sprinkle. It is, in most cases, quite unnecessary" (Lauren Bridges 2017).

I have found that in schools, nurseries and daycares people are not even waiting for the sniffle to arrive. They are prophylactically using essential oils every single day around our children. Blends containing clove, cinnamon, thyme thymol, oregano and eucalyptus are being used in small closed spaces without the informed consent of parents. As a parent of three children, I chose to make all the medical decisions for my child, whether it is using natural medicine or conventional medicine. It is not the place of teachers, administrators, daycare providers and nursery workers to make those decisions as to what each child is over-exposed to, let alone exposed to at all.

Best Practices with Babies, Children and the Elderly
Absolutely, *always*, dilute essential oils when using them with babies, children and the elderly. The permeability of skin, metabolism, medical history, contraindications and ability to process essential oils can be impacted by health, age, medications and size of the person using essential oils.

Essential Oils by Age		
Age	**Dilution rate**	**Considered Safe Essential Oils**
Premature + Newborn	0%	None
2-6 months	0.1%-0.2%	Roman Chamomile, Blue Chamomile, Lavender, Mandarin, Neroli, Geranium, Dill
7-12 months	0.25%-0.5%	Same as above and Tea Tree, Palmarosa, Petitgrain
2-5 years	1%-2%	Same as above and Ginger, Grapefruit, Vetiver, Tangerine

6-8 years	1%-2%	Same as above and Orange
9-11 years	Up to 2%	Same as above and Cypress, Eucalyptus
12+	2-5%	Same as above and otherwise check contraindications

Essential oils make the list of the top 25 substances most frequently involved in pediatric exposures in the 2016 American Association of Poison Control Centers report, with a whopping 13,972 exposures (American Association of Poison Control Centers 2016).

Not All Essential Oils Are Created Equal
You will find that contraindications are one of the most debated topics in the aromatherapy world. Some believe in erring on the side of caution, while others throw caution to the wind. Historically, many properties and contraindications given for essential oils are from herbal use and oral use, but the information is still very important. It is vitally important to understand that not all essential oils are created equal. The chemistry from oil to oil is vastly different. The entire topic of chemistry and a more in depth look at safety information is outside the scope of this book. If you would like to learn more about either topic I recommend reading *The Art, Science and Business of Aromatherapy*, 2nd edition by Kayla Fioravanti and *Essential Oil Safety*, 2nd edition by Robert Tisserand and Rodney Young and following the Essential Oil University on Facebook. For now here is an abbreviated review of the topic.

Know which essential oils to avoid or use with caution. Avoid them *even if* you like the way they smell or the properties that you read about them. The International Fragrance Association has a list of safety warnings regarding the use of essential oils. The warnings with only the more common essential oils listed include:

IFRA Banned Sensitizer: verbena.
IFRA Severely Restricted Oil: melissa.

IFRA Restricted Oils: oakmoss extracts, treemoss extracts, verbena absolute, and peru balsam.

IFRA listed Phototoxic/sensitizers: bergamot, bitter orange, lemon, grapefruit, lime, tangerine, mandarin, angelica root, clove leaf, and taget.

A Word About Wintergreen and Sweet Birch

I want to pause here and talk about wintergreen and sweet birch. Whether methyl salicylate is naturally occurring or synthetic, it has the risk of building up in the body and becoming toxic. Wintergreen essential oil naturally contains 98% methyl salicylate and sweet birch essential oil contains approximately 90% methyl salicylate. According to an article on Medscape, "One teaspoon of 98% methyl salicylate contains 7000 mg of salicylate, the equivalent of nearly 90 baby aspirins and more than 4 times the potentially toxic dose for a child who weighs 10 kg [22 lbs.]" (Muhammad Waseem 2017).

The common warnings for anything containing methyl salicylate or acetylsalicylic acid say that they must be avoided by people who have aspirin allergies, blood clotting disorders or are taking anticoagulant drugs. Additional warnings include those with asthma, history of seizures or epilepsy, those with fragile skin and connective tissue disorders, and those with a hyper-sensitivity to salicylates or who are pregnant or breast feeding. Exposure to methyl salicylate can cause Reye's Disease in children. Methyl salicylate may also raise red flags for those with congenital disorders, Ehlers-Danlos Syndrome, the elderly and purpura. Since it impacts blood clotting, anything containing methyl salicylate should be avoided altogether, before or after surgery. Wintergreen must absolutely be avoided by anyone taking blood-thinning drugs, since it increases the action of the drugs.

Health Canada restricts anything containing methyl salicylate to 1% for topical application. According to Clinical Advisor, salicylic toxicity can occur from an acute exposure or from lower doses taken over time, internally and topically. In 2009 there were more than 29,000 poison center reports of salicylic toxicity that resulted in 22 deaths (Fletcher Penney 2017).

The FDA has a specific regulation in place for wintergreen oil in which it warns, "Because methyl salicylate (wintergreen oil) manifests no toxicity in the minute amounts in which it is used as a flavoring, it is mistakenly regarded by the public as harmless even when taken in substantially larger amounts. Actually, it is quite toxic when taken in quantities of a teaspoonful or more. Wintergreen oil and preparations containing it have caused a number of deaths through accidental misuse by both adults and children. Children are particularly attracted by the odor and are likely to swallow these products when left within reach" (FDA). The FDA Code of Regulations Title 21 states that "the Department of Health and Human Services regards a product as misbranded if it contains more than 5% methyl salicylate (wintergreen oil) without a warning label" (FDA Code of Federal Regulations 2017). Unfortunately, for some reason, the multi-levels insist on ignoring safety recommendations about wintergreen and sweet birch. In the book, *Modern Essentials: A Contemporary Guide to the Therapeutic Use of Essential Oils* by Aroma Tools, "Application: Can be applied neat (with no dilution), or dilute 1:1 (1 drop essential oils to 1 drop carrier oil) for children and those with sensitive skin when used topically" (Aromatools). *Really? Suggesting neat and 1:1 dilution is reckless!* According to Tisserand and Young the maximum dermal dosage for an adult is 2.4%. And for a child—all the experts recommend that wintergreen and birch should not be used at all. A simple lick or taste of wintergreen can cause toxicity in a child 6 years or younger. For children 6 years and older a toxic dosage can be as little as 4 mL. Ingestion of 5 mL of wintergreen has caused deaths in children. Only 100 mg (0.0035 ounces) ingested over two days can produce toxicity. Repeated usage of wintergreen is extremely dangerous. "Mortality from chronic salicylate intoxication is considerably higher (25%) than from acute overdose (1 to 2%)" (Toxicology Data Network).

With so many amazing essential oils and the availability of Hemp CBD Oil to manage pain—why use wintergreen and sweet birch? It is too easy to unintentionally overdose on salicylates when one is unaware of exposure from various sources.

Go Forth and Use Essential Oils Safely

I have a confession to make. My natural medicine cabinet contains more than just essential oils. *Shocking, right?* How could a certified aromatherapist possibly turn to anything other than essential oils? Because after 20 years of aromatherapy experience, I know that essential oils are not the cure to everything. There isn't always *an oil for that*. Blasphemy! I know, but it's true. *This from a woman who sells essential oils and teaches aromatherapy?*

Yes—essential oils are amazing, wonderful, miraculous and healing—but they are not the answer to everything. My goal as an aromatherapist is to teach people how to safely use essential oils for a lifetime. I love essential oils, but believe it or not, there is more to my arsenal of natural remedies than aromatherapy.

My top five natural remedies include essentials oils, herbal medicine, fire cider, elderberry syrup, and hemp CBD oil. Other natural medicines that I recommend include: mushroom medicine, garlic honey, chiropractic care, acupuncture and homeopathy. Find a Nambudripad's Allergy Elimination Technique (NAET) practitioner near you if you have developed an allergy or hypersensitivity to essential oils. My family has had great success with NAET technique for allergy elimination—there are no guarantees, but certainly worth looking into.

We hope and pray that Stacey's story and my (Kayla) myth busting truths do not scare you away from essential oils. Our goal is to encourage you to become better educated by a wider group of experts—dive into the decades of research and training that is available nationally and internationally. We have included a recommended reading list and a list of online resources to help assist you as you expand your knowledge about essential oils. We encourage you to speak up, share your story and find support in your community, families, sphere of influence and especially in the *The Unspoken Truth About Essential Oils Facebook Group*. Help shine a light on the truth about essential oils.

EPILOGUE
by Sylla Sheppard-Hanger

Stacey is to be highly commended for the courageous act of sharing her own personal story through feelings, thoughts and pictures. With deep concern for others, Stacey had the desire to make her story public so that others can get the answers and help she did not. Kayla has done a great job of pulling in supporting information and resources to help those who may be experiencing some adverse effects from essential oils—or for those who wish to know what can happen, and what to do, if an adverse effect does occur. This book should be required reading in all aromatherapy schools and product sale classes before anyone recommends essential oils. My sincere hope is that by bringing this story to light, we can all become more aware and cautious of its uses. Besides the risk of overuse on the skin, overuse of essential oils is a waste of our precious resources, creating shortages and unsustainability.

I have been passionate about essential oils for 40 years, and during the 1980's, we saw the start of the new "EO Movement"—selling essential oils in a multi-level business model. Granted, this did introduce essential oils to the masses, but because of the lack of safety education and general safe practice knowledge not provided to users, this also created thousands of stories just like Stacey's. I recently realized that it's entirely because of this movement that my own path was set as I became a safety advocate and created my own movement, publicly standing up to this unsafe use. We quickly saw how these companies promoted the use of undiluted essential oils on the skin and cringed when they promoted drinking them in water. This misinformation spread quickly because the oils were used up faster, creating increased sales. This book is just one of hundreds of similar sad stories that I have witnessed over those years, both as past Chair of the now defunct NAHA safety committee, and as a collector of adverse effects and injuries reports collected on the Atlantic Institute of Aromatherapy site. The reports that are hosted on aromatherapyunited.org only represent a fraction of what is really happening.

I still find it a bit incomprehensible that a company portrays themselves as caring so much with good deeds to community, when they obviously do NOT care about their own user's health, only their continued sales. To brush off any adverse effects reported to them as detox or anomaly is hard to understand when we have had the information of safe use for over 50 years. Personally, to me it is even harder to understand how it has gone on this long without more lawsuits. Many people have suffered permanent damage, skin discoloration, continued and chronic issues, all due to bad information they received in good faith. I feel for the children who were dosed by well-meaning moms, who thought they were helping but hurt their own child. Only time will tell the number of scent aversions that have been created with the overuse of these precious oils.

I agree with Stacey that everyone in the company needs to be told what happened, instead of worrying about what may scare people off. In her words, "If people were more aware of what could happen to themselves or their children, they would understand just how powerful essential oils are and would hopefully use them like medications—only when needed."

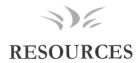

RESOURCES

Where to Report an Adverse Reaction

Atlantic Institute—AtlanticInstitute.com/injury-reporting/
Poison Control—Call (800) 222-1222
Tisserand Institute Adverse Reaction Database—
Tisserandinstitute.org/safety/adverse-reaction-database/

Online Resources

Alliance of International Aromatherapist—Alliance-aromatherapist.org

Aromahead Free Introductory Online Course—
Aromahead.com/courses/online

Aroma Medical—Aromamedical.org

Aromapologist—Aromapologist.com

Aromatic Plant Project—Aromaticplantproject.com

Aromatherapists Society—Thearomatherapistssociety.net

Aromatherapia Alliance—Aromatherapia.org

Aromatherapy Council—Aromatherapycouncil.co.uk

Aromatherapy Registration Council—Aromatherapycouncil.org

Aromatherapy United—Aromatherapyunited.org

Atlantic Institute of Aromatherapy—Atlanticinstitute.com

Canadian Federation of Aromatherapist—cfacanada.com

CBD (Hemp) Bio Care—CBDbiocare.com/yourinnerpiece (Stacey's affiliate link)

Crop Watch—Cropwatch.org

Essential Oil Analysis Foundation—Essentialoilanalysis.com

Essential Oil University—Essentialoils.org

Fioravanti, Kayla—Kaylafioravanti.com

Haluka, Stacey—YourInnerPiece.com

Hemp-Ology: Hemp-Ology.com (Kayla's Hemp CBD business)

International Federation of Aromatherapist (IFPA)—Ifaroma.org

International Fragrance Association—Ifraorg.org

International Journal of Clinical Aromatherapy—Ijca.net
National Association of Holistic Aromatherapist—Naha.org
Nambudripad's Allergy Elimination Technique (NAET) —Naet.com
Ology Essentials—OlogyEssentials.com (Kayla's essential oil business
& aromatherapy certification program)
Tisserand Institute—Tisserandinstitute.org
Tisserand, Robert—Roberttisserand.com
United Aromatherapy Effort—Unitedaromatherapy.org

On Facebook

Essential Oil Consumer Safety Advocates
Essential Oil University
The Unspoken Truth About Essential Oils
Tisserand Institute

Recommended Reading

Aromatherapy for Healing the Spirit: Restoring Emotional and Mental Balance with Essential Oils by Gabriel Mojay

Aromatherapy for Health Professionals, 4e by Shirley Price, Cert Ed FISPA MIFA FIAM; and Len Price, Cert Ed MIT (Trichology) FISPA FIAM

Aromatherapy Science: A Guide for Healthcare Professionals by Maria Lis-Balchin

Clinical Aromatherapy: Essential Oils in Practice, 2nd Edition
Author: Jane Buckle, PhD; RN–2003 (Advanced; Professional/Practitioner)

Essential Living by Andrea Butje

Essential Oil Safety: A Guide for Health Care Professionals, 2nd Edition by Robert Tisserand

Essential Oils and Aromatics: A Step-by-Step Guide for Use in Massage and Aromatherapy by Marge Clark

Essential Waters: Hydrosols, Hydrolats & Aromatic Waters by Marge Clark

Gattefosse's Aromatherapy: The First Book on Aromatherapy by Rene-Maurice Gattefosse (Edited by Robert B. Tisserand)

Holistic Aromatherapy for Animals by Kristin Leigh Bell

Hydrosols: The Next Aromatherapy by Suzanne Catty

Natural BabyCare: Pure and Soothing Recipes and Techniques for Mothers and Babies by Colleen K. Dodt

The Aromatherapy Book: Applications & Inhalations by Jeanne Rose

The Aromatherapy Practitioner Reference Manual by Sylla Sheppard-Hanger

The Aromatic Spa Book by Sylla Sheppard-Hanger

The Aromatic Mind Book by Sylla Sheppard-Hanger

The Art of Aromatherapy: The Healing and Beautifying Properties of the Essential Oils of Flowers and Herbs by Robert Tisserand

The Art, Science and Business of Aromatherapy: A Guide to Essential Oils & Entrepreneurship by Kayla Fioravanti

The Chemistry of Essential Oils: An Introduction for Aromatherapists, Beauticians, Retailers and Students by David G. Williams.

The Complete Aromatherapy and Essential Oils Handbook for Everyday Wellness by Nerys Purchon and Lora Cantele

The Complete Guide to Aromatherapy by Salvatore Battagia

The Essential Oils Book by Colleen K. Dodt

The Practice of Aromatherapy: A Classic Compendium of Plant Medicines and Their Healing Properties by Jean Valnet M.D.

375 Essential Oils and Hydrosols by Jeanne Rose

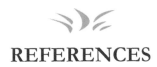

REFERENCES

American Association of Poison Control Centers. *2016 Annual Report of the American Association of Poison Control Centers' National Poison Data System (NPDS): 34th Annual Report.* November 29, 2017. Retrieved from https://aapcc.s3.amazonaws.com/pdfs/annual_reports/12_21_2017_2016_Annua.pdf

Aroma Tools. *Modern Essentials: A Contemporary Guide to the Therapeutic Use of Essential Oils.* Aroma Tools. 2008.

Aromatherapy United. *2017 Injury Reports Atlantic Institute of Aromatherapy.* PDF. Retrieved from http://aromatherapyunited.org/wp-content/uploads/2018/02/2017-Injury-Reports-Atlantic-Institute-of-Aromatherapy.pdf

Bauer, Kristina. *Essential Oils and the Detox Theory.* Tisserand Institute. June 18, 2015. Retrieved from http://tisserandinstitute.org/essential-oils-and-the-detox-theory/

Benton, Roxanne. Personal Communications. 2018.

Bridges, Lauren. *Risk vs. benefit: using potent antimicrobial essential oils with children.* Tisserand Institute. December 28, 2017. Retrieved from http://tisserandinstitute.org/antimicrobial-essential-oils-children/

Burfield, Tony and Sheppard-Hanger, Sylla. *Sensitization Revisited Again.* Atlantic Institute of Aromatherapy. Retrieved from https://atlantic-institute.squarespace.com/sensitization-revisited-again

Clymer, Melissa. *Facebook Post on The Unspoken Truth About Essential Oils.* February 27, 2018. Retrieved from https://www.facebook.com/groups/253055645202750/permalink/338632956645018/

English Oxford Living Dictionary. *Definition Inflammation.* Retrieved from https://en.oxforddictionaries.com/definition/inflammation

European Commission. *Introduction to Toxicology, Training for the Health Sector.* PDF. Retrieved from http://ec.europa.eu/health/ph_projects/2003/action3/docs/2003_3_09_a21_en.pdf

Farlex Partner Medical Dictionary. *Sensitization Definition.* Retrieved from https://medical-dictionary.thefreedictionary.com/sensitization

FDA Code of Regulations. *CFR-Code of Federal Regulations Title 21.* U.S. Food and Drug Administration. April 1, 2017. Retrieved from https://www.accessdata.fda.gov/scripts/cdrh/cfdocs/cfCFR/CFRSearch.cfm?fr=201.303

Fioravanti, Kayla. *The Art, Science and Business of Aromatherapy.* 2017. Selah Press. Franklin, TN.

Grand View Research. *Aromatherapy Market Analysis By Product (Essential Oils, Carrier Oils, Equipment), By Mode of Delivery (Topical, Aerial, Direct Inhalation), By Application, And Segment Forecasts, 2014–2025.* PDF Published Date: Aug, 2017. Retrieved from https://www.grandviewresearch.com/industry-analysis/aromatherapy-market

Hawkins. Beverley. *Skin Sensitization.* West Coast Institute of Aromatherapy. Retrieved from https://westcoastaromatherapy.com/articles/skin-sensitization/

International Fragrance Association. IFRA. *Annex I to the IFRA Standards (48th Amendment, June 2015).* PDF. Retrieved from http://www.ifraorg.org/Upload/DownloadButtonDocuments/4d5e6594-9c1b-4b10-b650-3abdc0e0134a/Index%20of%20IFRA%20Standards%2048th%20Amendment.pdf

International Fragrance Association. *IFRA Standards.* PDF. Retrieved from http://www.ifraorg.org/Upload/DownloadButtonDocuments/a13f9a09-ec56-4aab-a33b-ec66528d5330/booklet%20FINAL.pdf

Mayo Clinic. *Contact Dermatitis.* Retrieved from
https://www.mayoclinic.org/diseases-conditions/contact-
dermatitis/symptoms-causes/syc-20352742

Merriam Webster Dictionary. *Detoxify definition.* Retrieved from
https://www.merriam-webster.com/dictionary/detoxify

**Miller-Keane Encyclopedia and Dictionary of Medicine,
Nursing, and Allied Health.** *Sensitization Definition.* Retrieved from
https://medical-dictionary.thefreedictionary.com/sensitization

Mojay, Gabriel. *Aromatherapy entitled, British vs. French Aromatherapy—a
myth…or a smokescreen? An open letter to Sylla Sheppard-Hanger, Director of the
Atlantic Institute of Aromatherapy.* June 29, 2014. Retrieved from
https://www.facebook.com/notes/gabriel-mojay/british-vs-french-
aromatherapy-a-myth-or-a-smokescreen/1446399108944952/

Moore, Ginger. *Sensitization—What Is It and How To Reduce The Risk.*
Aromatherapy United. January 5, 2016. Retrieved from
http://aromatherapyunited.org/sensitization/

Mosby's Medical Dictionary. Sensitization Definition. Retrieved
from https://medical-dictionary.thefreedictionary.com/sensitization

Nelson, Ruth. *Facebook Post on The Unspoken Truth About Essential Oils.*
March 9, 2018. Retrieved from
https://www.facebook.com/groups/253055645202750/permalink/34
2916636216650/

Pappas, Robert PhD. *Myth #6.* Retrieved from
https://essentialoils.org/news/eo_myths/6

Penney, Fletcher. Salicylate toxicity. Clinical Advisor. Decision Sports
Medicine. 2017. Retrieved from
https://www.clinicaladvisor.com/hospital-medicine/salicylate-
toxicity/article/602872/

Peppermint Jims. When you think of mint, think of Peppermint
Jim's. Retrieved from http://peppermintjim.com/

Rhind, Jennifer Peace. *Essential Oils Handbook for Aromatherapy Practice*, 2nd edition. Page 18. Singing Dragon. 2012.

Rose, Jeanne. *Rose Oil—the many faces of a scent.* Jeanne Rose Aromatherapy and All Things Herbal. 2006. Retrieved from http://www.jeannerose.net/articles/RoseOil_manyfacesofascent.html

Taylor, Kelly Ann. *Facebook Post on The Unspoken Truth About Essential Oils.* February 27, 2018. Retrieved from https://www.facebook.com/groups/253055645202750/permalink/338632956645018/

The English Aromatherapist. *GRAS Essential Oils: Safe to Ingest?* Retrieved from http://englisharomatherapist.com/if-essential-oils-are-gras-are-they-safe-to-ingest/

Tisserand, Hana. *Grasse Phyt'Arom 2017–what we learned in France about French aromatherapy.* Tisserand Institute. October 25, 2017. Retrieved from http://tisserandinstitute.org/grasse-french-aromatherapy/

Tisserand, Robert. *Adverse Reaction Database.* Retrieved from http://tisserandinstitute.org/safety/adverse-reaction-database/#home/adverse-reaction-report-detailed-view/5996e998b34c36291baf0f98/

Tisserand, Robert. *Essential oils and eye safety.* February 23, 2013. Retrieved from http://roberttisserand.com/2013/02/essential-oils-and-eye-safety/

Tisserand, Robert. *New Survey Reveals Dangers of Not Diluting Essential Oils.* Updated December 13, 2017. Retrieved from http://tisserandinstitute.org/new-survey-reveals-dangers-of-not-diluting-essential-oils/

Tisserand Institute. *Adverse Reaction Database.* Retrieved from http://tisserandinstitute.org/safety/adverse-reaction-database/#home/adverse-reaction-report-detailed-view/5996e998b34c36291baf0f98/

Tisserand Institute. Safety Pages. *How to Use Essential Oils Safely.*

Tisserand Institute. Retrieved from
http://tisserandinstitute.org/safety/safety-guidelines/

Toxicology Data Network. Toxnet. *Salicylic Acid.*
https://toxnet.nlm.nih.gov/cgi-
bin/sis/search/a?dbs+hsdb:@term+@DOCNO+672

Watt, Martin. *Conclusions.* Aroma Medical. Aromamedical.org (please
do not share this link without written permission from Martin Watt)

Watt, Martin. Personal Communications. 2018.

Waseem, Muhammad, MBBS, MS, FAAP, FACEP, FAHA.
Medscape. *Salicylate Toxicity.* December 20, 2017. Retrieved from
https://emedicine.medscape.com/article/1009987-overview

ABOUT THE AUTHORS

Stacey Haluka

Stacey Haluka is Certified in Neuro-Linguistic Programming, Regression Therapy, Mindfulness, Reiki Energy Healing and as a Les Brown Motivational Speaker, Trainer and Transformational Coach. She is the Lead Shifter at Your Inner Piece and creator of Break Through, Break Free—Stacey is passionate about helping women create profound and permanent shifts through workshops, speaking engagements and one-on-one sessions.

Stacey believes that her painful experience with essential oils happened for a reason, so that she could help bring awareness to others. Since she had this experience, she has been blessed with a community of people who have supported her and wanted to help her heal. The knowledge and expertise passed on to her by the many essential oil experts is the reason this book has been written. Stacey is grateful for this opportunity to share her story. She hopes that it will encourage the reader to seek further training so that they will continue being blessed by the power of essential oils.

Kayla Fioravanti

Kayla Fioravanti is a certified aromatherapist, award-winning author and cosmetic formulator. In 1998, Kayla co-founded Essential Wholesale, which was listed as one of INC Magazine's 5000 Fastest Growing Companies in America three years in a row. Essential Wholesale began in Kayla's kitchen with a $50 investment in 1998 and sold for millions in 2011. Through Essential Wholesale, Selah-Press, Ology Essentials, private consultations, publications and public speaking, Kayla has literally been involved in thousands of businesses.

Kayla is a serial entrepreneur. After selling Essential Wholesale, she founded Selah Press in 2011, a one-stop-shop for book publishing and author coaching. On December 1, 2017, she launched Ology Essentials as an aromatherapy certification program and essential oils brand. At Ology Essentials, she also provides custom cosmetic formulating for companies of all sizes. Kayla also co-owns Hemp-Ology with her son Keegan and daughter-in-law Haleigh, which is a source for premium

Hemp CBD Oil and science-based information.

Kayla's books include: *The Art, Science and Business of Aromatherapy* (as well as a consumers edition called *The Art and Science of Aromatherapy*); *DIY Kitchen Chemistry*; *How to Make Melt & Pour Soap Base from Scratch*; *How to Self-Publish*; *Social Media: Platform Building Blocks for Both the Savvy & the Shy*; a memoir entitled *Puffy & Blue: The Chronicles of Nine Lives Together*; *360 Degrees of Grief*; a poetry book called *When I was Young I Flew the Sun Like a Kite* and a PDF book called the *Step by Step Guild to Self-Publish Using Createspace*.

Kayla lives in Franklin, Tennessee with her husband Dennis, their kids, along with cats, dogs, chickens and a herd of bison.

ABOUT THE CONTRIBUTORS

Dr. Robert Pappas

In 1996 Dr. Pappas worked as the senior chemist and perfumer for a well-respected essential oil and fragrance company. In 1998 he left his job to pursue a career as an independent consultant for the fragrance, flavor, and essential oil industry. Dr. Pappas started Essential Oil University in 1999 as a subscription database that was, and still is, the largest online database for the literature reference reports of GC/MS analyses of essential oils. Robert developed the first aromatherapy course to be offered for college credit in the U.S., as well as, the first college course on the chemistry of essential oils to be offered for credit at a state university. Out of the growing needs of his clients EOU became a supplier of essential oils to over 7000 small businesses, but his passion lead him back to full time consulting, analytical and educational company in 2011.

Providing unbiased analysis, accurate assessments, and unfiltered scientifically sound education are what companies large and small have come to rely on Dr. Pappas (commonly referred to as Dr. P) for. The Essential Oil Myths series on Essential Oil University has thoroughly disproved countless myths.

Robert Tisserand

Robert Tisserand is a speaker, educator and consultant on the science and benefits of essential oils and their safe and effective application. In recent years he has inspired live audiences in the UK, USA, Canada, Australia, Brazil, Czech Republic, China, Hong Kong, Taiwan, Korea and Japan on topics ranging from therapeutic action to the dynamic relationship between plant oils and the skin. Robert has 40 years of experience in aromatherapy "functional fragrance" product development. He was privileged to receive a Lifetime Achievement Award in Denver in 2007, and in 2014 he co-authored the second edition of *Essential Oil Safety*, a 780 page book published by Elsevier. Robert is the principal of The Tisserand Institute.

Martin Watt

Martin's expertise on the safety of using essential oils was developed over 25 years ago when he was asked to prepare safety guidelines by a UK aromatherapy oil suppliers association. Subsequently he created a trade safety manual, which went International and in addition to that he was consulted on safety issues by the largest UK pharmacy chain.

The safety information he assembled was partly based on published research of the USA based Research Institute of Fragrance Materials (RIFM) and their sister organization the International Fragrance Research Association (IFRA). Both organizations have a vast amount of experience and data on the use of essential oils. They are the main bodies advising the big International cosmetics and fragrance companies. My data sources were also drawn from the International dermatological publications where adverse reactions to substances are published. As well as a variety of medical adverse reaction reports going back over 100 years.

Martin was the first in the aromatherapy trade to investigate in any depth the great importance of skin reactions to essential oils and to publish that information. His publication *Plant aromatics* was on the market for 18 years until 2010, and sold copies around the word. Martin's particular interest has always been in finding scientific research that supports ancient healing knowledge, or rejecting traditional knowledge when this is proven inaccurate. That rejection of unsound knowledge has often bought him into clashes with those teaching it as fact, which has been common within the aromatherapy world.

Martin's accomplishments include, but are not limited to:

- Advisor on essential oils and aromatherapy to the Institute of Complementary Medicine - UK.
- Advisor on Education to the International Aromatherapists and Tutors Association in Canada.
- Taught aromatherapy classes in the USA, Canada and Korea, as well as trained visitors on private tuition courses.
- Has published several challenging articles in a number of aromatherapy publications and on the Internet.
- Compiled referenced research data suitable for medical professionals. Gave advice on treating leg ulcers, bed sores and infected cellulitis to a hospital in Scotland. This included the use of various essential oils and techniques for treating these

problems.

- Provided assistance and advice to a few aromatherapy authors and vetted training course materials.

- Advised companies on product development, and on issues of legislation regarding the sale of preparations containing botanical extracts.

- Co-authored the book *Frankincense and Myrrh* with Wanda Sellar. Now available in a kindle format.

All the above equipped Martin with an ability to judge the value or relevance of information, something rarely found in aromatherapy education. He is known in the aromatherapy trade for "not accepting they hype" and was well known on the newsgroups for fighting the purveyors of poor quality education and misinformation.

"I am detested by the many con artists in this trade, and loved by a few caring therapists. That's good enough for me." Martin Watt

Sylla Sheppard-Hanger

Sylla Sheppard-Hanger is the founder and director of the Atlantic Institute of Aromatherapy. In 1969, she became a Cosmetologist/Esthetician and a Natural Health Care Practitioner/Licensed Massage Therapist in 1978. She began teaching introductory through advanced studies of aromatherapy in 1988. In 1993, she completed the Medicinal and Aromatic Plants Program at Purdue University in Indiana. In 1997, she completed the International Training in Essential Oils: Advanced Studies. Sheppard-Hanger's book, *The Aromatherapy Practitioner Correspondence Course and The Aromatherapy Practitioner Reference Manual*, is a complete reference book of over 350 aromatic plant extracts, with phytochemical, clinical and botanical indexes.

Sheppard-Hanger was a founding member of the American Aromatherapy Association (1988) and served two terms on the Board of Directors. Sylla is an active participant in the National Association of Holistic Aromatherapy (NAHA) as Chair of the Safety Committee. She actively participates in setting up national standards in education for aromatherapy. She was a founding member and board member of the Aromatherapy Registration Council (ARC), which formed to promote the advancement of aromatherapy research and practice. Sheppard-Hanger founded the United Aromatherapy Effort, Inc

(UAE), a non-profit charity whose mission is collection and dissemination of donated aromatherapy products to those affected during critical incidents and emergency work during 9/11.

In 2014, Sheppard-Hanger began collecting essential oil injury reports in an effort to help the industry self-regulate before aromatherapy practices could become more regulated by governmental authorities, which could then limit the scope and range of essential oils for healing. Injury reports can be downloaded at AromatherapyUnited.org. Essential oil injuries can be reported at AtlanticInstitute.com. Sylla has played a vital role for decades in the field of aromatherapy and was recognized in 2017 by the Alliance of International Aromatherapists for Outstanding Contributions (Atlantic Institute).

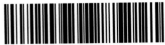

37171998R00049

Made in the USA
Columbia, SC
28 November 2018